THE HUMAN CANINE CONNECTION

Enriching Your Life by Loving Your Dog

DWAINE AJ WHOGOES

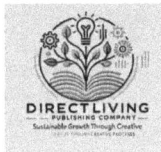

DIRECTLIVING
PUBLISHING COMPANY
Sustainable Growth Through Creative

Book Cover by Mr.TK
Illustrations by Dwaine AJ Whogoes
First edition 2024

Paperback - ISBN 9798332365669
Hardcover - ISBN: 9798332201776

ALSO BY DWAINE AJ WHOGOES

To the humans whose lives are enriched
To the dogs that put up with them
May we all live together in wellness
and with respect

TABLE OF CONTENTS

Introduction   11

1. DECODING DOG BEHAVIOR   15
   Dogs Are Complex Emotional Creatures   16
   The Science Behind Canine Emotions   16
   Recognizing Stress Signals in Dogs   19
   How Dogs Communicate: Understanding Canine
   Body Language   20
   The Role of Breed in Behavior and Temperament   23
   Puppy Psychology: Shaping Behavior From Young   25
   Senior Dogs: Adapting to Their Changing Needs and
   Behaviors   27

2. THE FOUNDATIONS OF DOG TRAINING   31
   The Heart of Training Our Dogs   32
   Positive Reinforcement: The Science and Art   32
   Setting the Stage for Successful Training Sessions   35
   Clicker Training Basics: Timing, Technique, and Tips   37
   Crate Training: Creating a Safe Haven   39
   The Essentials of Recall Training   41
   Mastering the Walk: Loose-Leash Training
   Techniques   43

3. BUILDING A STRONG HUMAN-CANINE BOND   47
   Building the Bond Through Playtimes   47
   The Power of Play: Strengthening Your Bond   48
   Reading Your Dog: Responding to Their Needs and
   Wants   51
   The Importance of Consistency in Relationship
   Building   53
   Trust Exercises: Building Confidence Together   55
   The Role of Touch: Massage and Physical Connection   58
   Shared Activities to Enhance Your Bond   60

4. ADDRESSING COMMON BEHAVIORAL
   CHALLENGES   63
   Barking Solutions: Understanding How Dogs
   Communicate and Reducing Noise   63
   Jumping Up: Training Your Dog to Greet Politely   66
   Dealing with Aggression: Strategies for Safety and
   Improvement   68
   Overcoming Separation Anxiety: A Step-By-Step
   Guide   70
   Leash Reactivity: Training for Calm Walks   72
   Resource Guarding: Prevention and Management   74

5. ADVANCED TRAINING TECHNIQUES   79
   Agility Training for Fun and Fitness   80
   Scent Work: Engaging Your Dog's Natural Abilities   83
   Trick Training: Strengthening Bonds Through Playful
   Learning   85
   Off-Leash Training: Steps for Success   87
   Behavioral Shaping: Modifying Complex Behaviors   89
   Therapy and Service Dog Basics: Training for a
   Purpose   92

6. THE HEALTHY DOG   95
   Nutrition's Role in Behavior   96
   The Impact of Exercise on Mental Health   98
   Recognizing and Addressing Pain in Dogs   101
   The Importance of Regular Veterinary Checkups   103
   Integrating Mental Stimulation into Daily Routines 105
   The Benefits of Routine and Structure   108

7. REAL-LIFE SUCCESS STORIES   111
   From Aggressive to Affectionate: A Rescue Dog's
   Journey   112
   The Senior Dog Who Learned New Tricks   114
   The Anxious Dog Who Found Calm   116
   A Journey of Trust: Rehabilitating a Fearful Dog   118
   Breaking Barriers: A Deaf Dog's Training Triumph   120
   The High-Energy Dog Who Became a Canine Good
   Citizen   123

8. BEYOND BASIC TRAINING 127
Canine Sports: Finding Your Dog's Passion 127
Dogs Giving Back: Volunteer and Therapy
Opportunities 130
The World From a Dog's Perspective: Enriching
Outings Seen Through Their Eyes 132
Canine Intelligence: How Dogs Think and Learn 134
Cognitive Training Games 135
Understanding Individual Learning Styles 135
Fostering Intellectual Growth 136
Innovations in Dog Training: Technology and New
Methods 137
Creating a Lifelong Learning Plan for Your Dog 140

Conclusion 145
References 149

INTRODUCTION

Dog ownership is a beautiful gift; people who discover a connection with the right dog are fortunate. I found great joy in raising my two pups, Joey and Hapa. My two Aussies traveled with me from the Coast of California to the Grand Canyon up and over the Rocky Mountains of Colorado. I have enjoyed watching them herd seagulls during off-leash walks along the West Coast, from San Francisco to Carmel by the Sea. They have traveled across the great Mississippi River on our way to Arkansas and endured sudden tropical floods driving through Oklahoma. Today, as we have grown older, we walk around our lake at home. Our bond, connection, and mutual adoration have been a lifelong journey of growing old and creating fond memories as good friends.

These furry creatures are more than just dogs; they are my family.

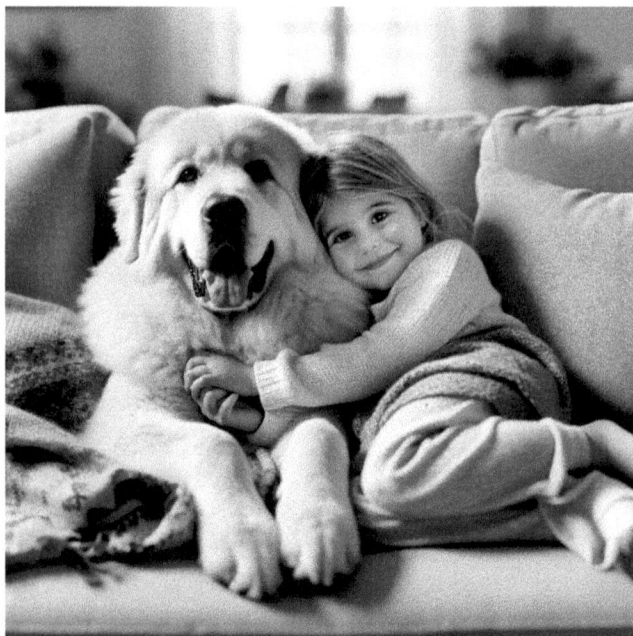

Have you ever felt that deep, unspoken bond as your dog gazes into your eyes as if peering into your soul? I remember those moments—a look, a head tilt, a wagging tail—that deepened my bond with my canine companion. These everyday interactions, laden with unspoken affection and loyalty, form the foundation of a profound yet unique relationship.

This powerful connection, woven from countless moments of joy, challenges, and companionship, illustrates our special connection with our canine friends. In these unguarded moments, we truly understand the emotional depth and complexities of the human-canine bond. This book is an ode to these moments and a guide to making them even more meaningful.

My name is Dwaine, and dogs have been my passion and faithful companions for as long as I can remember. From the muddy paws on the kitchen floor to the quiet comfort they offer in times of stress, my life's work has been to understand and enhance the connection between dogs and their human partners.

This book is born from a desire to share that lifelong journey with you—whether you are picking out your first puppy, trying to refine your training techniques, or simply seeking to deepen your bond with your canine companion.

In *The Human Canine Connection: Enhancing Your Life By Loving Your Dog*, I blend scientific insights with heartwarming stories and practical advice. This book is not just a guide; it's an invitation to explore the rich, emotional landscape you share with your dog. You'll find theories, methods, and interactive content that make this a hands-on experience.

What sets this book apart is its holistic approach. We delve into the latest research, offering a well-rounded understanding of your dog's behavior and needs. This book's research, real-life success stories, and practical training advice provide a comprehensive toolkit for fostering a thriving relationship with your dog.

This book is designed for everyone in the dog-loving community, from novices starting their journey to seasoned trainers looking for new insights. By acknowledging dog owners' diverse experiences and needs, I hope to provide a resource that is as inclusive as it is informative.

As we move through the chapters, you will be equipped with knowledge and the tools to apply this learning directly to your life. Expect to be engaged and challenged and to see your relationship with your dog transform.

The book is structured into distinct parts to guide your journey, each building on the last. Starting with foundational knowledge, we progress into practical training advice and delve deeper into how dogs perceive their world.

Let me share a brief story to give you a taste of what's to come. When I first met my dog Koa, he was a whirlwind of energy with little focus. You'll learn that through the methods in this book, Koa and I grew together, learning from each other. Today, he is calm and attentive and a true partner and friend. This transformation is what I hope to offer you.

So, are you ready to explore the depths of your connection with your dog and discover new ways to enhance this bond? Let's start this transformative journey together.

CHAPTER 1

DECODING DOG BEHAVIOR

Adopting a dog into a human family becomes an intricate part of that distinct family system. The two brothers discuss Marley, the family dog, in the following dialogue.

Marley is growing old and showing signs of illness, but he faithfully waits to greet his young friends at the local bus stop daily, as he has done for many years. When he hears the approaching bus, he runs to the mailbox to greet his two buddies as they return home from a long day at school.

"Is he there?"
"Of course, he's there; he's always there."
"How does he know we're coming?"
"Ah, I don't know, he just knows. Dogs know things like that."
"All dogs?"
"All good dogs."
"Oh, there he is! There's Marley!"
They step off the bus and onto the sidewalk. "Hi, Marley, how are you?"

"I missed you, buddy!"
(Grogan, 2009)

DOGS ARE COMPLEX EMOTIONAL CREATURES

Have you ever watched your dog sleep peacefully and suddenly start twitching or whimpering? Moments like these remind us that dogs are not just creatures driven by basic instincts but complex beings with emotions that often mirror our own. This chapter is about peeling back the layers of canine behavior to give you the tools to understand and empathize with your furry friend on a deeper level.

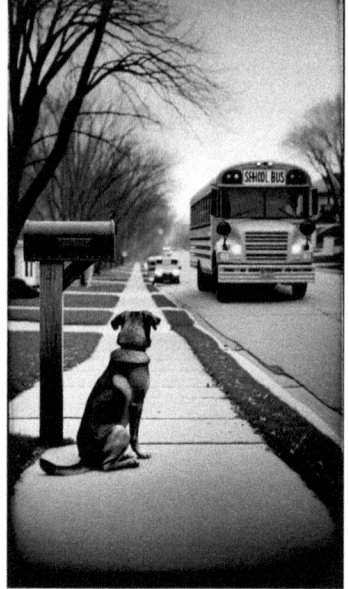

We often forget that our dogs experience a spectrum of emotions influencing everything they do, from that joyful sprint across the park to the anxious tuck of the tail during a thunderstorm. Understanding the science behind these emotions and learning to read the signs of their emotional well-being will allow you to foster a healthier, happier relationship with your dog.

THE SCIENCE BEHIND CANINE EMOTIONS

Emotional Intelligence in Dogs

Dogs have been our companions for thousands of years, and during that time, they have evolved to be extraordinarily attuned to human emotions. However, their emotional capacity is not just a reflection of ours; it is a rich tapestry that's wholly their own.

Research shows that dogs experience a range of emotions, including joy, fear, love, disgust, and even jealousy, in remarkably similar ways to humans. This emotional intelligence helps them navigate their social interactions and their environment in ways that maximize their well-being and survival.

For instance, when you pick up your dog's leash, and they start wagging their tail and spinning in excited circles, that is a joy—pure and unfiltered. On the flip side, if you have ever seen your dog slink away with its tail tucked after a scolding, you have witnessed its capability to feel shame or fear. These emotions are not just fleeting states but crucial for building the loyalty and affection bonds that make dogs invaluable companions.

Neurological Responses

What is happening in their brains during these emotional displays? Dogs share many of the same neurological structures that produce emotions in humans. The amygdala, for example, processes emotions like fear and pleasure by releasing hormones and neurotransmitters that prepare the body to react to various stimuli. When a dog feels threatened, their amygdala triggers a flood of stress hormones that lead to behaviors like growling or hiding. Conversely, positive interactions will activate the reward centers in their brains, releasing dopamine and encouraging them to repeat pleasing behaviors.

Understanding dog brain chemistry deepens our appreciation of their emotional complexity and enhances training strategies. By recognizing that specific training methods can cause stress or fear (as indicated by the dog's neurological responses), you can adjust your approach to use more positive reinforcement techniques that create pleasant associations.

Signs of Emotional Well-Being

Identifying the signs of a happy, healthy dog goes beyond noticing a wagging tail or an eager bark. Look for consistent eating habits, regular sleep patterns, playful behavior, and a general eagerness to interact with you and others. These signs often indicate that a dog feels secure and content in their environment.

Conversely, signs of distress or depression in dogs might be less obvious. Changes in behavior such as increased sleep, loss of appetite, avoidance of interaction, or unusual aggression can all indicate something is amiss. Like humans, dogs can experience mood shifts and emotional dips often triggered by environmental changes, health issues, or even shifts in household dynamics.

Influence of Emotions on Behavior

Every dog owner has witnessed how a dog's emotional state can directly influence their behavior. Fear can lead to aggression or submission, joy can lead to playful antics, and uncertainty can lead to anxiety-related behaviors such as excessive barking or chewing. Understanding these influences is crucial for responsible dog ownership. It allows you to create a supportive environment where your dog can feel secure and loved, reducing negative behaviors and enhancing your quality of life.

Recognizing and responding to your dog's emotional states lays the groundwork for a deeper, more empathetic relationship with your canine companion. This connection enriches your lives and forms the basis of practical training and mutual respect. As we continue to explore the nuances of dog behavior, remember that each wag, each whimper, and each gaze holds a wealth of information waiting to be understood.

RECOGNIZING STRESS SIGNALS IN DOGS

When your dog is stressed, it might not be as apparent as you think. Unlike humans, who can voice their anxieties, dogs communicate stress subtly. Recognizing these signs is crucial because prolonged stress can lead to health problems, behavioral issues, and a decreased quality of life for your furry friend. Let us start by understanding the common symptoms of stress in dogs. Excessive panting, drooling, and shedding are just the tip of the iceberg. You might also notice changes in their body posture—your dog may tuck their tail, lower their head, or flatten their ears. Some dogs may hide or display decreased activity, while others might do the opposite, showing restlessness or hyperactivity. These physical cues are your dog's saying, "I am not okay."

The triggers of these stress responses can be as varied as the dogs themselves. Loud noises like fireworks or thunderstorms are common culprits. Less apparent stressors, such as changes in the household, new environments, or even the absence of a family member, can also affect your dog. Separation anxiety is particularly prevalent among dogs, manifesting in behaviors such as destructive chewing, excessive barking, or attempts to escape. Each dog has its stress thresholds; what might be exciting for one dog could be terrifying for another. Understanding what stresses your dog is the first step in helping them cope.

Now, let's talk about calming techniques. The presence of a calm, reassuring human can work wonders. Simple actions like speaking softly and soothingly or gently petting can help alleviate stress. However, the effectiveness of these methods can depend on the dog's personality and the nature of the stressor. Creating a safe space in your home can provide a sanctuary from the stress of situations that involve separation anxiety or a fear of loud noises. This could be a quiet room away from the hustle and bustle of the household, outfitted with their favorite blanket or toy.

For long-term stress management, consistency is critical. Dogs thrive on routine as it gives them a sense of security. Keeping regular meals, walks, and bedtime schedules can help reduce anxiety. Environmental adjustments, like soundproofing your home during fireworks or providing interactive toys to keep them engaged while you're away, can also help manage stress. However, some cases might require professional help. Behaviorists can offer invaluable support, providing tailored strategies that address the root cause of the stress rather than just the symptoms. Behavioral therapy, environmental changes, and possibly even medical intervention can transform a stressed dog into a relaxed and happy companion.

Understanding and addressing canine stress is not just about improving behavior—it's about enriching our dogs' lives. They support us unconditionally with their companionship and love. Recognizing and alleviating their stress is one of the many ways to show our gratitude and ensure they lead happy, healthy lives. As we move forward, remember that each dog is an individual with unique needs and sensitivities. The journey to understanding and mitigating their stress is an essential step towards deepening the bond you share.

HOW DOGS COMMUNICATE: UNDERSTANDING CANINE BODY LANGUAGE

Have you ever wished you could ask your dog what was on their mind? While that might remain in fantasy, understanding your dog's body language can bring you surprisingly close to that. Dogs rely heavily on body movements, facial expressions, and vocalizations to express their feelings and intentions. By learning to interpret these signals, you can enhance communication with your canine friend, leading to a more harmonious and empathetic relationship.

Reading the Tail

The tail is like a dog's emotional barometer. Each wag, twitch, or droop can convey a different emotion or signal. For instance, a high, stiff tail often indicates alertness or aggression, particularly if it wags slowly. This is a sign that your dog is intensely focusing on something and might be assessing a potential threat. On the other hand, a relaxed tail held at mid-height suggests your dog is calm and comfortable with the situation. Excitement and happiness are usually displayed by a tail wagging vigorously. Conversely, a tail tucked between the legs clearly shows fear, submission, or anxiety. Watching how your dog's tail reacts in various situations gives you insight into their feelings, which can be especially useful in new or unfamiliar settings.

Facial Expressions and Vocalization

Dogs might not smile with their teeth like humans, but they still use their faces to express various emotions. Wide, bright eyes generally mean a dog is attentive and possibly excited. Narrowed eyes or a hard stare can indicate tension or aggression. It is essential to notice the context in which these expressions occur to understand their meaning entirely. Yawning might seem like a sign of tiredness, but it can also indicate stress or nervousness in dogs. Vocalizations also play a crucial role in communication. A high-pitched bark often signifies excitement or happiness, while a low growl could mean your dog is uneasy or threatening someone or something. Whining might be a request for attention or an expression of discomfort. By paying close attention to these cues, you can better understand your dog's immediate needs and emotional state.

Posture and Movement

The posture and movement of a dog can reveal a lot about their mood and intentions. A dog standing squarely on all fours, possibly slightly leaning forward, is typically alert and may be curious or somewhat cautious. A play bow—where the dog stretches its front legs forward, lowers its head, and keeps its rear end up—is an invitation to play and a sign of friendliness. Conversely, if a dog stiffens up and freezes, it may be a sign of discomfort or aggression. Understanding these postures and movements can help you predict and manage your dog's reactions, ensuring you both avoid potentially threatening situations.

Misinterpretations to Avoid

Misinterpreting canine signals can lead to miscommunications and even conflicts. For example, many people think that a wagging tail always means a dog is happy, but as we've seen, the nature of the wag can tell a different story. Another common misconception is that a dog baring its teeth is always an aggressive display. While this can be true, it might also be a submissive grin, a sign of anxiety, or an appeasement gesture in some contexts. Misreading these signals can lead to inappropriate responses from the owner, escalating rather than calming a situation.

You can foster a deeper understanding and a stronger bond by honing your ability to read and respond to your dog's body language. This communication forms the foundation of your relationship, enabling you to support your dog in any situation. As you become more adept at reading these cues, you'll find that your interactions with your dog become more fluid and natural, enhancing the joy and companionship that drew you to each other in the first place.

THE ROLE OF BREED IN BEHAVIOR AND TEMPERAMENT

When you're out at the dog park, do you ever notice how some dogs seem to sprint endlessly after Frisbees while others might be more content strolling around and sniffing every tree? Or perhaps you've seen a dog keen on herding the other dogs away from the park gates. These behaviors aren't random; they're often deeply rooted in a dog's breed-specific traits. Understanding these genetic predispositions is crucial because it shapes everything from their daily needs to the training approaches that resonate best with them.

Breed-Specific Traits

Each dog breed was initially bred for herding, hunting, guarding, or companionship. These tasks have left an indelible mark on these breeds' temperaments and energy levels. For instance, herding breeds like Border Collies or Australian Shepherds have a natural propensity for movement and may exhibit behaviors like circling or chasing. This is because they've been selectively bred for generations to herd livestock, requiring sharp reflexes and a high activity level. On the other hand, breeds like the Basset Hound were bred for hunting at a much slower pace, leading them to be generally more laid-back and less responsive to stimuli that might send a Border Collie into a tizzy.

Understanding these traits allows you to tailor your expectations and training to fit your dog's natural inclinations. If you own a high-energy breed, you should invest in more mentally stimulating toys and activities. A more reserved, gentle training approach might be necessary for a naturally timid breed like the Greyhound.

Understanding Prey Drive

Prey drive is another breed-specific characteristic that significantly impacts behavior. This instinctual behavior is seen in the dog's inclination to chase and capture smaller animals and is particularly strong in breeds like Greyhounds and Huskies. It's a highly valued trait in hunting breeds, making them excellent at tracking and catching game. However, in a modern living environment, high prey drive can manifest as chasing smaller pets, bolting after squirrels during walks, or focusing intensely on moving objects like cars or bikes.

Managing a dog with a high prey drive requires consistent, focused training to help them control their impulses. It also means providing them with appropriate outlets for this drive, such as lure coursing or flirt pole activities, which can satisfy their chase instincts in a controlled, safe environment. Understanding this aspect of your dog's behavior is vital in preventing incidents and ensuring their energy is channeled positively.

Socialization Needs

The level of socialization a dog requires can also be influenced by its breed. Socialization involves exposing your dog to various experiences, environments, and individuals to ensure they are well-adjusted and comfortable in different situations. Breeds that are naturally more suspicious of strangers, like many guard dogs, will benefit from more intensive, positive exposure to various people and settings to prevent the development of fear-based aggression. Conversely, breeds known for their sociability, like Labrador Retrievers, may be more forgiving of less frequent socialization but still benefit from regular interactions to maintain their friendly disposition.

Proper socialization involves more than just exposure; it requires creating positive experiences. For sensitive breeds, this might mean gradual introductions to new environments and plenty of treats and praises to build positive associations. For more outgoing breeds, it is vital to ensure they learn appropriate social behaviors, like not jumping up on strangers or overwhelming other dogs.

Training Considerations

Finally, it would be best to consider your dog's breed-specific traits when deciding how to train it. High-energy breeds capable of quick, agile movements, like the Border Collies above, often excel in fast-paced training environments involving many movements, such as agility courses or advanced obedience. These activities channel their energy and satisfy their need for mental stimulation and physical exercise. In contrast, breeds with lower power and more independent nature, such as Chow Chows, might respond better to training that involves shorter, highly engaging sessions that respect their more aloof nature.

Adapting your training methods to suit your dog's natural tendencies makes training more enjoyable for both of you and increases the likelihood of success. It's about working with their nature, not against it, and recognizing that each breed has something unique. This tailored approach guarantees that your training efforts are met with enthusiasm and better outcomes, fostering a deeper bond and mutual respect between you and your dog.

PUPPY PSYCHOLOGY: SHAPING BEHAVIOR FROM YOUNG

When discussing raising a puppy, we often focus on the immediate: house training, basic commands, and social manners. However, what's equally crucial—and perhaps even more impactful in the long run—is understanding and guiding the psychological development of a young dog during what's known as the critical social-ization period. This period, typically the first three to four months of a puppy's life, is when they are most open to new experiences and learning about the world around them. The impressions and lessons learned during this time can profoundly influence their behavior into adulthood.

Think of it this way—every interaction, experience, and reaction they witness is a building block in the foundation of their future self. This is when a puppy learns whether the world is safe or scary, which creatures are friends and which are foes, and how to react in various situations. Neglecting the importance of this period can lead to a dog with behavioral issues such as fear, aggression, or anxiety. Conversely, a well-socialized puppy is typically more confident, outgoing, and stable.

For new dog owners, understanding the significance of this window of opportunity is the first step. The next, naturally, is applying this knowledge through foundation training techniques that foster obedience and confidence. Simple practices like positive reinforcement can be incredibly effective. This method rewards good behavior—such as sitting, staying, or coming when called— with treats, praise, or play, reinforcing the behavior you want to see without punishment. It encourages your puppy to associate obedi-ence and good behavior with positive outcomes, making them more likely to repeat these behaviors.

Moreover, it's crucial to address potential behavioral issues preemptively. This proactive approach involves recognizing early signs of undesirable behaviors, like resource guarding or excessive barking, and nipping them in the bud through gentle correction and redirection. For instance, if a puppy starts to growl when someone approaches their food bowl, it's a teachable moment. You can work on desensitization by approaching the bowl and adding better treats. And because they eat, this gradually helps them understand that the approach of a human to their food bowl is a joyous event, not a threat.

Encouraging curiosity and play is an essential part of a puppy's development. Play not only burns off excess energy. It's also critical for their cognitive and emotional development. Through play, puppies learn problem-solving skills, improve their motor skills, and understand the rules of social interaction with other dogs and humans. Toys like puzzle feeders that stimulate their minds can be particularly beneficial. These not only entertain them but also teach them patience and persistence. Similarly, playing with your puppy can strengthen your bond and help them learn appropriate behaviors in a fun, stress-free environment.

Remember that each puppy is unique, and what works for one might not work for another. This individual variability means that while the principles of puppy psychology are universal, their application should be tailored to suit each puppy's personality and learning style. Observing and adapting to your puppy's responses during the critical socialization period can lead to a well-adjusted, happy adult dog, making the effort during these early days well worth it. As we explore the nuances of canine development and behavior, remember that your journey with your puppy lays the groundwork for a lifetime of companionship and mutual understanding.

SENIOR DOGS: ADAPTING TO THEIR CHANGING NEEDS AND BEHAVIORS

As our canine companions enter their golden years, they begin to show signs of aging, just like humans do. It's a natural process, but it often comes with challenges that can affect their behavior and overall well-being. Recognizing these age-related changes is vital in ensuring our senior dogs live happy, comfortable lives even as their needs evolve.

One of the most noticeable changes in aging dogs is an increase in anxiety or confusion. This can often be attributed to the decline in their cognitive functions, a condition sometimes referred to as Canine Cognitive Dysfunction, which is akin to dementia in humans. Signs might include disorientation, changes in sleep patterns, less interaction with family members, or even forgetting commands they once knew. It's heart-wrenching to witness, but understanding that these are symptoms of a deeper issue can help us respond with patience and empathy.

As your dog's senses wane—perhaps their hearing isn't what it used to be, or their vision is fading—they might startle more easily or become anxious in situations that previously didn't bother them. This heightened anxiety can sometimes lead to increased vocalization; your once quiet companion might now bark at the slightest noise. Maintaining a routine that gives them a sense of security and predictability is essential to keep their living environment as stress-free as possible. Minor adjustments, like keeping their bed in a quiet corner away from high-traffic areas or maintaining a consistent schedule, can make a difference in their comfort.

Adjusting care for their comfort involves daily routines and the physical environment. As dogs age, their mobility decreases, and they might find it hard to navigate around the house. Ramps or steps can help them access their favorite couch or bed without straining their joints. Non-slip mats can prevent falls on slippery floors, and extra bedding can cushion aging bones. Also, consider the height of their food and water bowls; raising them can ease the strain on their neck and back.

Maintaining mental health in senior dogs is just as crucial as addressing physical limitations. Keeping their mind engaged can slow the progression of cognitive decline. Simple activities, adapted to their pace, can stimulate their brain and keep them engaged. Puzzle feeders are great for encouraging mental activity, requiring them to solve simple problems with their food. Short, gentle training sessions can keep their minds sharp, reinforcing basic commands or teaching new, low-impact tricks that don't strain their aging bodies.

Navigating health issues in senior dogs means being vigilant and proactive. Watching for signs of discomfort or pain that might affect their behavior is vital. Limping, reluctance to jump or use stairs, increased lethargy, or even changes in how they carry their tail— often a sign of pain in the lower back or hips—can all indicate underlying health problems. Regular veterinary checkups become increasingly important as dogs age, as early detection of issues like arthritis, dental disease, or organ failure can drastically improve their quality of life.

When you notice changes in your dog's behavior or mobility, consult your vet. They can offer treatments such as medications for arthritis or supplements that support cognitive function. Sometimes, changes in diet can help manage weight, reduce stress on aging joints, and provide the nutrients necessary to support an older dog's health. Remember, each dog ages differently, and what might be right for one senior dog might not suit another. The goal is always to tailor your care to meet your companion's specific needs.

As our senior dogs slow down, we must adjust our lives to fit their pace. They might not be able to go on long hikes or play fetch for hours like they used to, but they still enjoy the sun's warmth during a short walk or the comfort of sitting by our side. It's a time to repay the loyalty and love they've shown us through the years, ensuring their twilight years are filled with comfort and joy. Watching a dog age isn't easy, but with the proper care and attention, their senior years can be satisfying, filled with moments of gentle companionship that underscore the enduring bond between humans and their canine friends.

CHAPTER 2

THE FOUNDATIONS OF DOG TRAINING

D ogs are as dear to us as our human children. I once heard a story about a dog that was found sitting on the front porch of its old master's new home. The owner had been moved to a nursing facility across town several miles away, and the animal followed his master's scent to his new home.

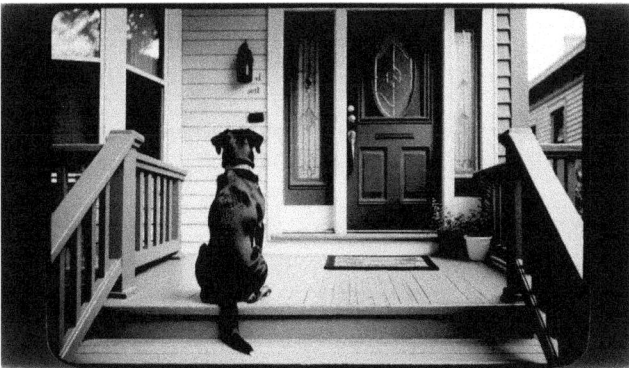

Our longing for this "homeward bound" scenario is unique yet profound. So, let us continue to explore this deep affection we share with our dogs. The emotional bond between our species demonstrates our innate need for faithful companionship and unbridled love.

THE HEART OF TRAINING OUR DOGS

Imagine you're teaching a toddler to speak. You would celebrate each correctly pronounced word and gently guide them through their mistakes, right? Training your dog is similar. It's about communication, patience, and positive reinforcement. This chapter dives into the heart of dog training, starting with a method that's as effective as it is kind: positive reinforcement. This approach strengthens the bond between you and your dog and fosters an environment of mutual trust and respect—critical ingredients for any successful training regimen.

POSITIVE REINFORCEMENT: THE SCIENCE AND ART

Principles of Positive Reinforcement

Positive reinforcement is a cornerstone of modern dog training, deeply rooted in psychological principles. At its core, it's about rewarding behaviors you want to encourage, thereby increasing the likelihood that these behaviors will be repeated. It's based on the law of effect, a theory by psychologist Edward Thorndike that states that actions followed by pleasant consequences are likely to be repeated, while those followed by unpleasant consequences are not.

(Thorndike, 1911)

When applied to dog training, this means rewarding your dog with treats, praise, or play whenever they perform a desired behavior. This could be as simple as sitting when asked or as complex as navigating an agility course. The reward makes them more likely to repeat the behavior in the future, effectively shaping their actions over time.

Implementing Reward Systems

The effectiveness of positive reinforcement hinges on the reward system you use. Rewards can vary widely depending on what motivates your dog. Some dogs may do a happy dance for a piece of kibble, while others might prefer a quick game with a favorite toy or verbal praise. The key is to find what best motivates your dog and use it consistently as a reward.

It's also important to vary the rewards to prevent boredom and maintain your dog's interest in training. While food is a common and powerful motivator, integrating play and affection ensures that your dog doesn't just obey the treat but also enjoys the process, strengthening your bond.

Timing and Consistency

Timing is critical in positive reinforcement. The reward must be given within seconds of the desired behavior. This helps the dog make a clear connection between the behavior and the reward. If there's a little delay, your dog might not associate the reward with the correct action, slowing down the learning process.

Consistency is equally important. Every time your dog performs the desired behavior, they should receive a reward. This consistency helps reinforce the learning and makes the training process quicker and more effective. It's also crucial that everyone in your household follows the same training guidelines. Consistency across different trainers provides clear and steady learning cues, which helps prevent confusion and mixed messages.

Avoiding Common Pitfalls

While positive reinforcement is a highly effective training method, it has its pitfalls. One common mistake is inadvertently rewarding the wrong behavior. For example, if you give your dog a treat to stop them from barking, they might learn that barking leads to treats rather than quiet behavior. Being mindful of what behavior you are reinforcing with your rewards is vital.

Another pitfall is overreliance on treats. While treats are a powerful motivator, they shouldn't be the only tool in your training arsenal. Integrating other rewards, such as toys, play, and praise, can make training more engaging for your dog and prevent it from becoming dependent on food rewards.

Finally, inconsistency in training can undermine your efforts. If you only enforce rules sporadically, your dog might learn that rules are optional. Consistently enforcing commands and boundaries clarifies what is expected of your dog, leading to better overall obedience and a happier, more secure dog.

Interactive Element: Reflection Section

Take a moment to think about what motivates your dog the most. Is it treats, toys, or perhaps praise? How can you incorporate these motivators more effectively into your training sessions to ensure they are engaged and responsive? Reflecting on these questions can help you tailor your approach to fit your dog's unique personality and needs, making your training sessions more effective and enjoyable for both of you.

In the following sections, we'll explore how to set the stage for successful training sessions, delve into the specifics of clicker training, and more. Each segment builds on the last, equipping you with a comprehensive toolkit to help your dog learn and thrive. As we move forward, remember that dog training is not just about teaching commands—it's about fostering a deep intimacy and understanding connection with your canine companion.

SETTING THE STAGE FOR SUCCESSFUL TRAINING SESSIONS

Creating the right environment for dog training is like setting up a classroom for young students—it needs to be conducive to learning, free of unnecessary distractions, and tailored to foster focus and positivity. Imagine trying to teach a skill in the middle of a bustling street compared to a quiet, secluded park; the setting undeniably impacts the ability to concentrate and absorb information. For dogs, this means finding a space where both of you can be relaxed without interruptions. A quiet room in your home or a peaceful corner in your yard can serve as perfect training grounds. Check that the area is safe and enclosed, especially if your dog is still learning to respond to recall commands. Remove any distractions that might divert your dog's attention from you, such as toys scattered around or other pets and people walking about. However, remember that the goal isn't to isolate your dog but to minimize excessive stimuli that could hinder their ability to focus on the tasks.

Setting realistic goals for each session is crucial once you've established a suitable training environment. It's easy to dream of your dog mastering a new command in a single session, but real progress is usually more incremental. Start by setting small, achievable objectives for each session, which could be as simple as improving a sit command's duration by a few seconds or getting one step closer in a multi-step trick. Acknowledge every small victory and use it as a building block for more complex tasks. This approach keeps you realistically grounded and provides a sense of accomplishment for you and your dog, making the training sessions enjoyable and rewarding. Remember, the ultimate goal is gradual improvement, not instant perfection.

Engagement and motivation are the fuel of practical training sessions. Dogs, much like humans, vary in what keeps them interested and eager to learn. While some dogs might find a particular treat irresistible, others might be more driven by verbal praise or a quick play session. Keep your sessions dynamic and unpredictable by rotating the rewards and incorporating games into the training process. This makes learning fun and keeps your dog guessing, which can heighten their interest and engagement. For instance, after a successful recall, instead of immediately handing out a treat, you might engage in a brief tug-of-war, which can be a powerful motivator for many dogs. Also, be mindful of your energy and demeanor during training; dogs are incredibly perceptive and can easily pick up on your emotions. A cheerful, energetic attitude from you can inspire the same in your dog, making training more effective.

Lastly, an effective session structure is critical to maximizing learning and retention. Each training session should have a clear beginning, middle, and end. Start with a warm-up using your dog's commands to get them into a "working" mindset. This reinforces previous learning and boosts their confidence as they start with something familiar. Then, introduce new material or focus on a skill you wish to develop. Keep this segment short to maintain concentration, especially for puppies or highly energetic dogs with shorter attention spans. Conclude with a cool-down period, revisiting more manageable tasks, or playing a relaxing game to end on a positive note. This structure keeps training sessions concise and focused and helps your dog learn to transition in and out of training mode, which can be beneficial in everyday situations where you need them to listen and respond quickly.

By meticulously crafting the training environment, setting attainable goals, keeping your dog engaged, and structuring sessions for optimal learning, you create a foundation for practical and enjoyable training. This facilitates faster learning and strengthens the bond between you and your dog, making each session something both of you can look forward to. As we move forward, remember that each dog is unique, and what works for one might not work for another. The key is to be observant, adaptable, and responsive to your dog's needs and responses, ensuring that your training methods evolve along with your growing relationship.

CLICKER TRAINING BASICS: TIMING, TECHNIQUE, AND TIPS

Imagine you could communicate with your dog through a simple, consistent sound that says, "Yes, that's exactly what I wanted you to do!" That's what clicker training accomplishes. This method uses a small handheld device that produces a sharp, quick sound—a "click"—to communicate precisely when your dog does something correctly. The beauty of clicker training lies in its simplicity and effectiveness. It uses the principles of operant conditioning, focusing on reinforcing behaviors you want to see repeated, and it does so clearly and immediately, making it easier for your dog to understand and follow.

The clicker's sound cuts through the noise of everyday life and tells your dog that whatever they were doing at that exact moment was right and will earn them a reward. The consistency of the click sound as a marker helps speed the learning process. It's more distinct and immediate than verbal praise, which can vary in tone and timing, potentially confusing your dog. With clicker training, your dog hears the same sound every time they perform correctly, creating a strong association between the behavior and the reward that's about to come. This method affects a dog's confidence during training sessions and their eagerness to learn, as they clearly understand their expectations.

Mastering the use of a clicker is crucial to the success of this training technique. The first step is ensuring that the click is always followed by a reward, typically a treat, solidifying the click-reward connection in your dog's mind. Begin with simple commands your dog knows, such as "sit" or "stay." When your dog executes the command, click and immediately offer a treat. This precise timing helps your dog associate the click with the desired behavior and the following treat. You can use the clicker to shape and refine new behaviors as you progress. The key is consistency and timing; the click must happen when your dog does what you want, followed quickly by a reward.

As your dog becomes more attuned to the clicker, you can increase the complexity of your training behaviors. This could involve combining learned behaviors into sequences or gradually introducing more challenging tasks. For example, if your dog has mastered sitting when asked, you might move on to having them sit at a distance or sit with increasing distractions around. The clicker can help you fine-tune these behaviors, such as clicking for slight improvements or holding a seat longer than before. It's like shaping clay; each click sculpts your dog's behaviors and understanding, gradually molding their actions into your desired form.

However, as with any training method, you might encounter challenges when starting with clicker training. One common issue is the timing of the click, which might only sometimes sync perfectly with the desired behavior. This can lead to confusion if the click sounds too early or too late. Suppose you find this happening; practice timing without your dog by clicking at specific moments while watching a video of dogs performing behaviors. Another challenge is over-reliance on clickers and treats, which can become a crutch if not gradually phased out. Start reducing the frequency of clicks and treats as your dog becomes more consistent. Instead of clicking every single time, begin to click for only the best executions of the behavior or introduce variable rewards, where not every click leads to a treat.

Clicker training offers a fun, rewarding way to communicate with your dog, bolsters their learning, and strengthens your bond. It turns training into a game where every click brings a sense of achievement, and every treat is a well-earned prize. As you and your dog become more proficient in this method, you'll find that the clicker can help you work through even the most complex of behaviors, enhancing your dog's skills and your relationship.

CRATE TRAINING: CREATING A SAFE HAVEN

Crate training, often misunderstood as confining or restrictive, is one of the most effective tools in your dog training arsenal, providing a multitude of benefits both for you and your furry companion. At its heart, crate training cultivates a personal space for your dog to feel secure and relaxed, much like their own room. This sense of security is vital, especially in a bustling household or during stressful situations like thunderstorms or large gatherings. It's important to remember that dogs innately seek out small, den-like spaces to rest and recharge; hence, a crate naturally aligns with their instinctual needs. Beyond comfort, crate training is crucial in-house training, as dogs typically avoid soiling their sleeping quarters. This helps establish and maintain a straightforward routine for bathroom breaks, significantly easing the house-training process.

Introducing your dog to a crate should be a gradual and positive experience. Start by selecting a crate that allows your dog to stand up, turn around, and lie comfortably. Please place it in a common area of your home where they can still feel a part of the family activities, as isolation can lead to stress and anxiety. Add a soft bed and some favorite toys to make the crate inviting. Begin by encouraging your dog to explore the crate with the door open, using treats to create positive associations. Feed meals near the crate initially, then place the food inside, allowing your dog to enter and exit freely. Gradually increase your dog's time in the crate with the door closed during and after meals. If they appear relaxed, try creating them briefly while you're home, slowly extending the time as they grow more comfortable.

Navigating crate training effectively involves knowing what to do and what to avoid. Always ensure that the crate remains a positive space. Never use it as a punishment, as this can create negative associations and anxiety around the crate. While letting a puppy out when they whine about being confined is tempting, it can reinforce the idea that crying is the way to get out, potentially leading to problematic behaviors. Instead, wait a moment before opening the crate to reinforce calm behavior. Also, be mindful of what is left in the crate with your dog; avoid items that could be chewed up and swallowed, posing a choking hazard or causing intestinal blockages.

Balancing crate time is crucial to ensure it benefits your dog without becoming excessive. While crates are valuable for managing behavior and safety when you can't supervise your dog, they are not meant to replace proper exercise and interaction. Dogs shouldn't spend all day in a crate. Give your dog ample time outside the crate to move, play, and bond with you and your family. For adult dogs, a general guideline is no more than four to five hours at a time in the crate, with puppies needing even more frequent breaks to stretch and relieve themselves. If your schedule requires your dog to be crated longer than this, consider incorporating a dog walker or a pet sitter to provide relief during the day.

Incorporating these practices helps transform the crate into a haven your dog respects and appreciates as a personal retreat. As crate training progresses, many dogs seek out their crate voluntarily, valuing its tranquility. This transition not only underscores the effectiveness of the approach but also highlights how a proper introduction and the balanced use of a crate can enrich your dog's life, providing them with a secure space entirely on their own.

THE ESSENTIALS OF RECALL TRAINING

When you think about letting your dog roam in the park or even wander off-leash on a trail, the first thing that might come to your mind is, "Will they come back when I call?" That's where mastering the art of recall—or teaching your dog to return to you upon command—becomes valuable and essential for safety. Having a reliable recall means that in potentially dangerous situations, such as near a busy street or in the presence of a threatening animal, you can trust your dog to return to you swiftly when called. This skill can be a lifesaver, making it one of the most important commands your dog should learn.

Building a solid foundation for recall begins in environments where distractions are minimal. Start indoors or in a fenced yard where competing stimuli are controlled. The goal is to make returning to you the best option available to your dog every time. Use a happy, enthusiastic tone to call your dog to you, pairing the command with their name, like "Fido, come!" Ensure that every time they come to you, it results in a positive experience. High-value treats, a favorite toy, or heaps of praise and affection should immediately follow their compliance. This consistent positive reinforcement makes the act of coming when called a rewarding experience for your dog, reinforcing the behavior you want to see.

Once your dog reliably responds to the recall command in a low-distraction setting, it's time to up the ante. Gradually introduce more challenging environments to the practice, such as a park with other people and dogs at a distance. It's crucial to incrementally increase the difficulty level to keep your dog successful at each stage. If your dog fails to come when called at any point, it may mean you've moved too fast in the training process. Returning to the last environment where they were successful, reinforce the behavior before trying again. Using a long leash during this stage of training can help you manage and gently guide your dog's responses without escalating into a chase.

Even with the best training, recall challenges can arise, and knowing how to handle these bumps in the road can make a big difference. One common issue is the dog becoming selectively deaf to the recall command when something more interesting catches their attention. This selective hearing can be frustrating and is often a sign that your training sessions must be more engaging or rewarding. Reevaluate the rewards you are using—are they high value enough to compete with the distractions your dog faces? Additionally, playing the "recall game" can inject fun into the train-ing. Call your dog back and forth between two people, rewarding them each time they come to you. This reinforces the command and turns it into a stimulating game.

Another issue might be the overuse of the recall command, leading to it becoming background noise to your dog. If you call your dog repeatedly without a response, it's time to reduce the distance, reduce distractions, and gradually build up again. Remember, every call should have a purpose, and your dog's triumphant return should be met with substantial rewards. By keeping each recall event positive and rewarding, you make sure that your dog won't start tuning out what could be the most crucial word they ever need to heed.

Incorporating these strategies will enhance the safety of your outdoor adventures with your dog and deepen the trust and bond between you. As you continue to build on these recall fundamen-tals, remember that patience and consistency are your best tools for crafting a reliable response. Each step forward in recall training is a step towards more freedom and enjoyment in the many adventures you and your dog will have together.

MASTERING THE WALK: LOOSE-LEASH TRAINING TECHNIQUES

Walking your dog should be a pleasurable experience, not a tug-of-war. Yet enthusiastic canine companions pull many dog owners down the street. Teaching your dog to walk on a loose leash is essential for enjoyable, stress-free outings and is foundational to good leash manners. When your dog learns to walk without pulling, it allows for safer interactions and better control, particularly in public spaces where distractions abound.

Loose-leash walking is simple: Your dog walks calmly by your side with the leash hanging in a "U" shape without tension. This skill is crucial for your dog's comfort and for fostering a respectful relationship where you lead and your dog follows. The benefits extend beyond mere convenience; it reinforces your role as the pack leader and teaches your dog self-control and focus, which are beneficial in various aspects of life.

The right tools and equipment are vital to begin training for loose-leash walking. While traditional collars can work for dogs that don't pull, a no-pull harness is a kinder option for those that do. These harnesses typically attach at the chest, redirecting your dog's attention towards you when they start to pull without causing strain on their neck and throat. It's important, however, to choose a harness that fits well to avoid discomfort and ensure it functions as intended. Additionally, a fixed-length leash offers more control than retractable ones, which can inadvertently encourage pulling by always keeping tension on the leash.

Training your dog to walk on a loose leash is a gradual process that requires patience and consistency. Start in a quiet environment with minimal distractions, like your backyard or a seldom-used park. Begin by letting your dog explore freely on a leash to burn off some initial excitement and energy. Once they're calmer, start your training. Every time your dog pulls, stop walking immediately. Stand still and wait until the leash relaxes. You can also change direction and reward your dog when they catch up and walk beside you again. These techniques teach your dog that pulling gets them nowhere while walking calmly by your side moves them forward.

Distractions are the most significant challenge when it comes to mastering loose-leash walking. Other animals, people, moving vehicles, and exciting smells can all entice your dog to forget their training. To maintain focus, practice attention exercises. Before you walk, spend a few minutes on simple commands like "sit" or "look at me." Rewarding these behaviors with treats or praise helps reinforce that listening to you is more rewarding than any distraction. Gradually introduce more distractions into your training sessions. This might mean walking near a busy park or down a street where you'll encounter other dogs. Keep your training sessions short and positive, and end them before either of you get frustrated.

By integrating these techniques and maintaining consistency, you'll find walking more enjoyable and less chaotic. It's a gradual process, but with persistence, your dog will learn that walking calmly on a leash is the best way to move forward, literally and figuratively.

Reflection Section: Interactive Element

Take a moment to observe your next walk: What are the main distractions causing your dog to pull? How do you react when pulling occurs? Reflecting on these questions after your walk can help identify specific challenges and adjust your training strategy accordingly.

As we wrap up this chapter, remember that training your dog in any capacity, whether recalling or walking nicely on a leash, is about building a relationship based on mutual respect and understanding. The techniques discussed here are stepping stones to creating a bond that enhances obedience and enriches your companionship with your dog.

In the upcoming chapter, we'll explore more advanced training techniques that challenge your dog and introduce fun and engaging ways to strengthen the skills they have learned so far. From agility training to therapeutic tasks, you'll discover how to keep your dog mentally stimulated and eager to learn, ensuring their training continues to be a rewarding experience for both of you.

CHAPTER 3

BUILDING A STRONG HUMAN-CANINE BOND

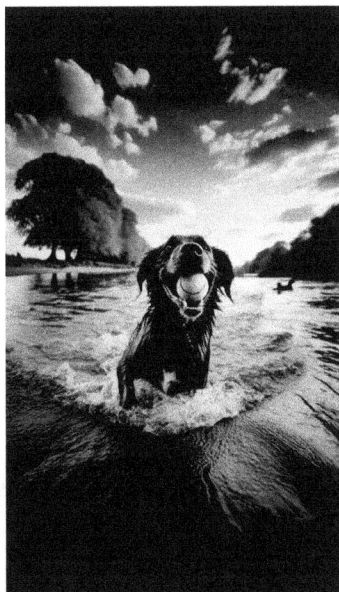

G od created dogs to satisfy man's basic need for companionship. Dogs reduce stress and relieve emotional pain.

Dogs play significant roles in the homes of millions of families today, which may be indicative of why we allow them prominence in our lives. I think the human-canine relationship is rich, powerful, and simply unique.

BUILDING THE BOND THROUGH PLAYTIMES

Bonding with your dog is not just about spending time together; it's about making each moment count. Often seen as mere fun, play is a part of building and strengthening the bond between you and your dog. It's a way to communicate love, establish social rules, and enhance mutual understanding while having a great time together. Playing also provides mental stimulation and physical exercise, which are critical to your dog's well-being. Through playful interactions, you reinforce training, boost confidence, and deepen the trust between you and your canine companion, making every game you play together an investment in your relationship.

THE POWER OF PLAY: STRENGTHENING YOUR BOND

Play as a Bonding Tool

Imagine tossing a ball in a park and watching your dog chase it with unfettered joy—their tail wagging, eyes bright, and an unmistakable smile spreading across their face. This simple activity, while entertaining, is also a powerful tool in reinforcing the bond you share. Play creates a shared language of joy and cooperation that transcends the basic owner-pet dynamic, fostering a deeper connection. During these moments of shared excitement and fun, proper bonding occurs, breaking down barriers and building trust. Moreover, play sessions are perfect opportunities to integrate training naturally and enjoyably. Commands like "come," "sit," "stay," or "drop it" can all be woven into fun activities, reinforcing these behaviors in a positive, relaxed environment. This improves your dog's obedience and enthusiasm for learning as the lines between play and training blur in an engaging, educational experience.

Types of Play and Their Benefits

Play can take many forms, each with distinct benefits. Fetch, for example, enhances a dog's agility and responsiveness while providing a great physical workout. Tug-of-war, often misunder-stood, is a fantastic way to teach self-control and strengthen your dog's muscles—if it's played with clear rules like "let go" or "drop it" on command. Puzzle toys require a dog to solve a problem, engage their minds, and hone their problem-solving skills to receive a reward. Each type of play engages different aspects of your dog's personality and abilities, contributing to a well-rounded, satisfied, and well-behaved pet. The correct play can also depend on your dog's age, health, and temperament. Puppies may burst with energy and enjoy more vigorous play, while older dogs might prefer gentler, more strategic games that don't strain their joints.

Training as Play

Integrating training into play is about making learning fun and natural. Use games to reinforce commands and good behavior. For instance, during a game of fetch, use the moment when your dog brings the ball back to practice "sit" or "stay." This reinforces the commands and teaches your dog to control their excitement, a valuable skill in various social situations. Similarly, hide-and-seek can enhance a dog's "come" command training. Start by asking your dog to stay, hide somewhere nearby, and then call them to you. Reward them with lots of praise and a treat when they find you. These playful training sessions boost your dog's skills and eagerness to participate, making training something they look forward to.

Safety Guidelines for Play

While play is beneficial, keeping it safe and positive is crucial. Always supervise play sessions, especially when new toys or games are introduced. Ensure the toys are appropriate for your dog's size and chew strength to avoid any risks of choking or accidental ingestion. Be mindful of the physical limits of your dog; intense play should be balanced with periods of rest to prevent overexertion, especially in hot weather. Watch for signs of frustration or aggression during play—sometimes dogs get overly excited or possessive, and it's important to recognize when to calm things down. Establishing rules like stopping the game if it gets too rough teaches your dog to play gently and safely, ensuring that playtime remains a positive bonding experience.

Interactive Element: Play and Reflect

After your next play session, take a moment to reflect on how you might use play more effectively as a training tool. Consider what types of games your dog enjoys most and how you might subtly use those preferences to reinforce training commands. Could a game of tug-of-war help with teaching "drop it"? Might a fetch session extend their patience and improve their "stay" ability? Reflecting on these questions can help you turn everyday play into powerful learning opportunities, enhancing the bond you share with your dog while enriching their life and yours.

By understanding and utilizing the power of play, you enrich your dog's life and foster a deeper, more trusting relationship. This chapter sets the stage for further exploring how everyday interactions can enhance the bond you share with your canine companion. Reading your dog's body language and following consistent training practices can improve your bond with your canine companion. Through thoughtful engagement and a bit of creativity, play can become a cornerstone of a loving, respectful relationship filled with joy and mutual understanding.

READING YOUR DOG: RESPONDING TO THEIR NEEDS AND WANTS

Understanding your dog goes beyond teaching them commands and managing their daily routines; it involves tuning into their non-verbal cues and comprehending their emotional states. Every tail wag, ear twitch, or subtle shift in posture has meaning; learning to interpret these signals can deepen your bond. Dogs communicate primarily through body language; each gesture or expression can provide insights into their feelings and needs. For instance, a relaxed posture and soft eyes usually indicate contentment, while a tucked tail and lowered head might suggest fear or anxiety. By staying observant and responsive to these cues, you create a deeper understanding and trust between you and your dog, paving the way for a more harmonious relationship.

To effectively respond to your dog's needs, it's crucial to recognize the subtleties of their behavior. This awareness allows you to address issues before they escalate into more significant problems. For example, if you notice your dog licking their lips and yawning, these could be signs of stress in specific contexts. Recognizing these early signs allows you to remove your dog from stressful situations, preventing anxiety. Similarly, if your dog suddenly starts barking at a new object in the home, acknowledging their alertness and then calmly introducing them to the object can help alleviate their fear, showing them there's nothing to worry about.

Meeting your dog's emotional needs is as important as meeting their physical ones. Like humans, dogs feel a wide range of emotions, and understanding these emotions can help you respond more effectively to their needs. When dogs feel understood, they are more likely to feel secure and attached to their owners. Emotional support might involve comforting a dog scared of loud noises during thunderstorms or giving a nervous dog extra space and time to warm up to strangers. Addressing these emotional needs, you help your dog cope with their immediate feelings and foster a sense of safety and trust that strengthens your bond.

Anticipating behavioral needs is another integral aspect of reading your dog. This proactive approach involves understanding potential triggers and knowing how your dog might react in different situations. Suppose your dog becomes overexcited and jumps on guests. You can anticipate and manage this behavior by having them on a leash as guests arrive, redirecting their energy with a toy, or practicing sit-stays. By anticipating and managing these situations, you prevent unwanted behaviors from becoming habitual, making your dog more straightforward and pleasant.

Respecting individuality plays a pivotal role in how you interact with your dog. Each dog has a unique personality shaped by genetics, upbringing, and experiences. Some dogs may be outgoing and adventurous, while others are reserved and cautious. Understanding these differences is critical to providing the proper support and training tailored to their needs. For example, an adventurous dog might thrive on hiking adventures that allow them to explore, while a more cautious dog might prefer quiet walks in familiar surroundings. By acknowledging and respecting these preferences, you ensure your dog's happiness and well-being and reinforce their trust in you as someone who truly understands them.

Reading and responding to your dog effectively hinges on understanding their communication methods, emotional needs, and personality. This understanding fosters a supportive environment where your dog feels valued and understood, deepening your bond. It's about building a relationship that goes beyond the surface, rooted in mutual respect and empathy, where you and your dog are attuned to each other's needs and preferences. As you continue to develop this skill, you'll find that your interactions with your dog become more fluid and intuitive, leading to a more rewarding and fulfilling relationship.

THE IMPORTANCE OF CONSISTENCY IN RELATIONSHIP BUILDING

Consistency in training and the application of rules are the bedrock upon which the trust and security of a dog-human relationship are built. Imagine if you lived in a world where the reactions and expectations of those around you changed unpredictably from one moment to the next. This would likely lead to feelings of confusion and insecurity. For dogs, whose understanding of the world depends heavily on the predictability of their environment and their humans' behavior, consistency is not just comforting—it's crucial.

Consistent rules and training methods guide your dog in navigating their world confidently. When dogs know what is expected of them and that following these expectations leads to positive outcomes, they are much more likely to feel secure and exhibit desirable behaviors. This doesn't just apply to fundamental commands like sit, stay, or come but also to your responses to their actions. For instance, if jumping up is met with laughter and petting one day and a stern reprimand the next, it creates confusion, making it harder for your dog to learn the appropriate way to greet people.

Routine and predictability play significant roles in creating a comforting environment for your dog. Dogs thrive on routine because it makes the world predictable and less threatening. Regular feeding times, walks, and play periods help structure your dog's day, giving them a sense of order and security. A stable routine can be particularly beneficial for dogs who suffer from anxiety. It reassures them that despite whatever uncertainties exist in the world, their basic needs will be met consistently. Consider, for example, a rescue dog from an unstable environment. Establishing a predictable routine can be instrumental in helping them adjust to their new home. Knowing when they will eat, walk, and spend time with you can alleviate stress and build the trust they need to settle in and bond with you.

Clear and consistent communication is crucial in deepening your bond with your dog. This involves not only the consistency of commands but also the consistency of your emotional responses and the methods of communication you choose. Dogs are highly perceptive and can pick up on subtle cues in body language and tone of voice, which can sometimes speak louder than words. If your verbal commands are inconsistent with your body language, it can confuse your dog. For example, telling your dog to come while leaning away from them might be interpreted as a sign to stay back. Ensure your signals, commands, and body language are aligned and consistently used to foster understanding and compliance. This clarity helps your dog understand your expectations and learn appropriate behaviors more quickly.

Building trust through reliability is one of the most critical aspects of developing a deep, trusting bond. Dogs look to their owners for guidance and reassurance. Being a reliable figure in their lives strengthens their trust in you. This means being dependable in providing for their basic needs and being emotionally present for them. When a dog learns they can rely on you to protect, lead, and care for them, their trust in you deepens, and their dependence on you for security becomes steadfast. This trust is vital not only for building a strong bond but also for practical training. A dog who trusts its owner is likelier to follow commands, even in distracting or stressful situations, because it believes that following your lead will keep it safe and secure.

You create a framework of trust and security that underpins a robust and lasting relationship with your dog through consistent training, a predictable routine, clear communication, and reliability. Through this framework, your bond can grow, rooted in mutual respect and understanding, allowing you both to navigate the complexities of life with confidence in each other. As you continue to build this consistency into every aspect of your interactions with your dog, you'll find that the trust and connection between you do not just enhance your training efforts but enrich your lives together.

TRUST EXERCISES: BUILDING CONFIDENCE TOGETHER

Building trust with your dog is akin to weaving a tapestry—intricate, requires attention to detail, and every thread counts. Trust-building exercises are those threads, each one designed to strengthen the bond and confidence between you and your canine companion. These activities are not just about teaching tricks or commands; they're about creating a foundation of mutual respect and understanding that can transform your relationship. For example, a simple "find the treats" game can do wonders. Hide treats around your house and encourage your dog to find them. This game stimulates their mind and places you as the source of fun and rewards, deepening their trust in you.

Another effective trust-building exercise is the "obstacle course" game. Set up a simple course at home with cushions, boxes, or outdoor furniture. Lead your dog through the course gently. This activity helps build physical confidence and reinforces your role as a guide and protector, showing your dog that they can rely on you in unfamiliar or challenging situations. The key here is to encourage and praise them for every little success, no matter how small, whether they navigate a new obstacle or overcome a hesitant moment. This boosts their confidence and cements their trust in your leadership.

Overcoming Fears Together

Helping your dog overcome their fears is critical to building a trusting relationship. Fear can be a significant learning barrier and affect your dog's well-being. The approach here is gentle and gradual exposure to the source of fear, paired with positive reinforcement. Suppose your dog fears loud noises like thunder or fireworks. You could start by playing recordings of these sounds at a low volume during happy times like meals or play. Gradually increase the volume over several sessions, ensuring your dog is comfortable and relaxed. This method, known as desensitization, helps them associate the once-fearful noise with positive experiences, reducing their anxiety.

Another common fear is meeting new people. If your dog tucks their tail or growls when someone new comes into the home, it's a clear sign of anxiety or discomfort. To help them overcome this, ask friends to help with a cheerful greeting routine. Have them approach slowly, avoiding direct eye contact, and offer a treat or a toy. This changes the narrative around strangers from a threat to a bearer of good things. Remember, your dog's comfort level should always dictate the pace. Forcing too much too soon can reinforce fear, so patience here is your best tool.

Building Trust with Patience

The role of patience in building trust cannot be overstated. Every dog learns and adapts at their own pace, and recognizing this is crucial in developing a solid bond. It's like learning to dance; you wouldn't expect to get the steps right immediately—it takes practice and patience. The same goes for your dog. They may not understand what you're asking of them right away, or they may struggle with a particularly frightening experience. In these moments, your calm, patient presence is reassuring. It tells your dog they are safe and there's no rush; you're in this together for as long as it takes. This assurance is foundational in building trust.

For instance, if you're training your dog to stay alone at home without anxiety, start with very short periods of separation and gradually increase the time. If they start getting anxious, it means you've moved too fast. Step back. Shorten the separation time again, moving slowly to build their confidence. Throughout this process, your patient, supportive approach teaches your dog that they can trust you consistently to return, thus easing their anxiety.

Celebrating Small Victories

Recognizing and celebrating small victories is essential in trust-building efforts. Every small step your dog takes towards overcoming a fear or learning a new skill is a milestone in the trust-building journey. It's these small successes that pave the way for more significant achievements. For instance, the first time your dog allows a new person to pet it without cringing or the first time they stay calm during a thunderstorm are victories that should be celebrated. These celebrations, whether extra treats, enthusiastic praise, or more playtime, reinforce positive behaviors and make your dog feel loved and valued. They also remind you of your progress, which is essential because trust-building can sometimes be slow and challenging.

In your day-to-day interactions with your dog, look for these small victories. Maybe they didn't pull on the leash as much today, or perhaps they managed to sit still for a few seconds longer than yesterday. Acknowledge these moments with a smile, a loving pat, or a cheerful word. This reinforces the behavior and strengthens your emotional connection, fostering a deep, enduring bond built on mutual trust and respect. Through these trust exercises, you create an incredibly fulfilling relationship with your dog rooted in a deep understanding and respect for one another.

THE ROLE OF TOUCH: MASSAGE AND PHYSICAL CONNECTION

The touch of a hand can speak volumes, especially to a dog whose language of love and comfort often lies in the physical connection they share with their human. Petting your dog helps cement your bond and affects their emotional and physical health. When you stroke your dog's fur, scratch their favorite spot, or engage in gentle massage, you're doing more than just showing affection; you're activating a cascade of beneficial hormonal responses that can improve their well-being and deepen the trust in your relationship.

Many animals, including dogs, need touch to feel an emotional connection. Regular, gentle physical contact can reduce stress and anxiety and improve physical health. Studies have shown that when dogs are petted, their bodies release oxytocin, the same hormone that helps bond mothers with their babies (Pet Science Daily, 2021).

This hormone plays a significant role in bonding and helps to increase trust and peacefulness. Additionally, physical contact lowers cortisol levels, the stress hormone, which can help make your dog feel more relaxed and at ease. This hormonal exchange not only benefits your dog but can also elevate your mood and reduce your stress levels, creating a mutual benefit that is truly heartwarming.

Introducing the concept of canine massage can take this connection even further, transforming your touch into a powerful tool to enhance your dog's health and deepen your bond. Massage for dogs is like massage for humans, involving gentle, rhythmic stroking and kneading of the muscles that can help increase circulation, relieve muscle tension, and promote better relaxation. Start with your dog in a calm, comfortable position, and use a soft touch to slowly stroke along their body, following the direction of their fur. Please pay attention to how they respond to different pressures and areas, adjusting your touch accordingly. Focus on places like the neck, shoulders, and back, avoiding sensitive spots like the belly and paws unless your dog is comfortable.

While regular massage and touch benefits are great, observing and respecting your dog's comfort levels with physical contact is key. Not all dogs are comfortable with the same types of touch or being touched in all areas. Due to past injuries, some might be ticklish or have sensitive spots in certain places. It's essential to watch for signs of discomfort, such as pulling away, panting, licking lips, or flattening ears. These signals are your dog's way of setting boundaries. Respecting these signals by adjusting or stopping touch prevents stress and reinforces their trust in you. You need to be attentive to their needs and respect their limits.

The therapeutic benefits of touch extend beyond emotional well-being and into physical health. Regular massage can help detect early signs of health issues, such as lumps, bumps, or areas of sensitivity that may require veterinary attention. For older dogs, gentle massage can help alleviate the pain and stiffness associated with arthritis, improving mobility and quality of life. Regular massage can help reduce the risk of injuries for active dogs by enhancing muscle flexibility and circulation.

Incorporating touch into your daily routine with your dog can transform routine petting into an impactful tool for emotional and physical healing. It strengthens your bond, providing comfort and security to your dog while offering you a peaceful, intimate way to care for their well-being. As you continue to explore the power of touch, remember that each stroke, each gentle press, and every moment of physical connection is a building block in the loving relationship you are nurturing with your canine companion.

SHARED ACTIVITIES TO ENHANCE YOUR BOND

Selecting suitable activities to share with your dog can turn simple daily routines into cherished moments that emphasize your connection. The key here is to choose activities you and your dog find enjoyable, ensuring that the time spent together strengthens your bond. For instance, hiking might be a perfect way to spend quality time together if you love the outdoors and your dog has a good amount of energy. On the other hand, if you're more of a homebody, engaging in interactive games like hide and seek indoors can be just as bonding. The goal is to find common ground where your interests meet, creating enjoyable and enriching experiences for both of you.

The bonding power of shared experiences with your dog cannot be overstated. These activities do more than pass the time; they build trust, enhance communication, and strengthen your emotional connection. Every new adventure or shared activity serves as a building block for a stronger relationship. For example, when you and your dog navigate a new trail together, overcome a challenging obstacle, or even learn a new game, you create memories and experiences reinforcing your bond. These shared experiences also help build your dog's confidence and can reduce anxiety by providing positive interactions with the world around them.

When it comes to bonding activities, variety is vital. Exploring new environments is particularly enriching for dogs as it stimulates their senses and provides exciting new challenges. Activities like hiking provide physical exercise and expose your dog to different smells, sights, and sounds, which can be mentally stimulating. Whether done formally or improvised in your backyard with homemade obstacles, agility training can also be a fun and rewarding way to spend time together. It engages your dog's mind and body while reinforcing skills like obedience and quick learning. Even more straightforward activities like visiting a new dog park or taking a different route on your walk can introduce elements of novelty and excitement into your dog's life.

Incorporating daily bonding moments into your routine is crucial for maintaining and enhancing your connection with your dog. These don't have to be time-consuming or elaborate; even small interactions can make a big difference. For instance, maintaining a routine where your dog helps you pick up the morning newspaper can turn an ordinary task into a special daily ritual. Similarly, ending each day with a calm cuddle or a gentle grooming session can help you unwind and reinforce the feeling of safety and companionship. These moments, though brief, remind your dog of their valued place in your life, and they show that bonding doesn't need to be reserved for special occasions—it can be part of the fabric of your everyday life.

Engaging in shared activities is about more than just having fun together; it nurtures a relationship that offers both of you emotional support, security, and joy. You create a deep, enduring bond that enriches every aspect of your life when you choose activities that suit both personalities, embrace the power of new experiences, and find joy in the little moments. By exploring new activities and integrating these bonding moments into your daily routine, you'll find that your relationship with your dog grows more robust and more fulfilling because it is anchored in mutual love and respect.

As this chapter closes, we reflect on how structured play, consistent interactions, and thoughtful engagement contribute to a robust, loving relationship with our canine companions. These efforts are not just about training or managing an animal; they're about honoring the connection that makes dogs such memorable parts of our lives. Looking ahead, we'll explore advanced training techniques that challenge your dog and enhance the skills and bonds developed through these foundational activities.

CHAPTER 4

ADDRESSING COMMON BEHAVIORAL CHALLENGES

I recently heard a story about a dog in Moore, Oklahoma, who was found by the county sheriff's department covered in mud, sitting amidst the rubble where a tornado had demolished an entire community. At first, it was thought the pup was just another

miracle among all the scattered rubble. But later, rescuers realized the dog was guarding the remains of its deceased owner buried beneath the debris. (Huffington Post, 2013).

BARKING SOLUTIONS: UNDERSTANDING HOW DOGS COMMUNICATE AND REDUCING NOISE

Isn't it fascinating how a dog's bark can sometimes seem like a language

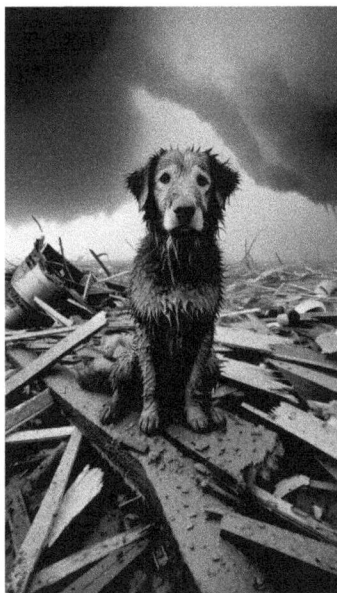

all its own? Each bark can hold a
wealth of information, whether it consists of excited yips when you
grab the leash or low, wary growls as a stranger approaches the
door. Understanding this canine communication can increase your
connection with your furry friend and help them navigate the
world more peacefully. This chapter delves into common yet often
misunderstood barking behavior, equipping you with the knowledge and strategies to manage it effectively, ensuring a quieter and
happier household.

Identifying Causes of Barking

Barking is a natural dog behavior and a primary mode of communication. However, excessive barking can be challenging for dogs
and their families, often signaling underlying issues that need
addressing. Broadly, barking can be categorized into a few types:
attention-seeking, alarm, boredom, and reactive.

Attention-seeking barking occurs when a dog has learned that it leads
to human interaction, whether positive or negative. This type can
often be inadvertently encouraged by owners responding to their
dog's barking with attention, even if it's to scold them. *Alarm
barking* is triggered by perceived threats, like someone approaching
the house—it's your dog's way of alerting you and warding off
potential intruders. *Boredom barking* usually results from a lack of
mental and physical stimulation. It's a dog's saying, "I'm bored and
need something to do!" Lastly, *reactive barking* is seen in dogs
responding to specific stimuli in their environment, like another
dog passing by the yard.

Understanding the root cause of your dog's barking is the foundation for addressing it effectively; observing when and where it
barks can give you valuable clues about what's driving its behavior.
Is it when they're left alone? When do they see another animal

outside? When the doorbell rings? Identifying these triggers is necessary to manage the behavior appropriately.

Training Alternatives to Barking

Training your dog to respond to a "quiet" command is a powerful tool to manage excessive barking. This training teaches your dog that silence can be as rewarding as barking. Start by choosing a command or signal—like "quiet" or a hand signal—and use it consistently whenever your dog barks inappropriately. When your dog ceases barking, immediately reward them with a treat or praise, even for just a few seconds. Over time, extend the duration of silence required before the reward comes. Remember, with patience and consistency, you can see significant improvements in your dog's behavior.

Positive reinforcement is essential here; it encourages your dog to associate silence with positive outcomes and strengthens the bond between you and your pet. Consistency in training, as with all types of dog training, is crucial. It might also be helpful to train an incompatible behavior—a behavior that can't be done while barking, like holding a toy in their mouth. This stops the barking and redirects their energy into something positive.

Environmental Management

Adjusting your dog's environment can reduce unnecessary barking. For example, if your dog barks at stimuli outside the window, managing their access to windows or using visual barriers like curtains can help. If the barking is due to boredom, increasing their physical and mental stimulation can make a big difference. This could involve more walks, playtime, and puzzle toys that challenge their minds. The goal is to address the needs that barking is misguidedly trying to fulfill. Rest assured, these strategies have been proven effective in numerous cases, and with your dedication, you can create a more peaceful environment for you and your dog.

Consistent Response

Ensuring that everyone in your household responds to your dog's barking similarly is vital to managing the behavior effectively. Mixed responses can confuse your dog and make the problem worse. Establish household rules for responding when dogs bark and ensure everyone sticks to them. This consistent response helps your dog learn appropriate behaviors more quickly and effectively.

Interactive Element: Reflection Section

Take a moment to think about the last time your dog barked excessively. What were the circumstances? Reflecting on what might have triggered the barking and how you responded can help you understand what changes might be needed, either in your dog's environment or your responses to their barking.

Understanding and managing barking is more than just silencing unwanted noise—it's about responding to your dog's needs and emotions to respect their natural behaviors while maintaining a peaceful home. As we continue exploring common behavioral challenges, remember that each behavior is an opportunity to learn more about your canine companion and enhance the bond you share.

JUMPING UP: TRAINING YOUR DOG TO GREET POLITELY

When your dog greets you or a guest with a leap up to your chest, it's often a sign of unbridled joy and excitement. Understanding why dogs jump up helps redirect this enthusiasm in a more socially acceptable manner. Dogs jump up because face-to-face greetings are standard in their pack-based social structure and denote affection and greeting. Puppies jump up to lick the faces of returning mother dogs as a welcome and to stimulate regurgitation of food. While this behavior is natural, it's not always appreciated by humans, especially when the enthusiastic greeter is a full-sized adult dog. Training your dog to keep all four paws on the ground during greetings makes interactions safer and more pleasant.

Reward your dog whenever they greet someone without jumping to teach the desirable "four on the floor" behavior. You can do this through positive reinforcement techniques such as treats, praise, or petting. The key is to reward them immediately when all four paws are on the ground, ideally before they even think about jumping. If your dog starts to jump, turn away and ignore them until they calm down and their paws return to the floor. Consistency is vital here. Every time your dog greets someone, the same rules must apply. Over time, your dog will learn that keeping all four paws on the ground is the quickest way to earn your affection and attention.

Offering an alternative greeting can also help manage your dog's enthusiasm. Training your dog to sit or lie down when someone enters the home effectively channels their excitement into a calm, controlled action. Begin by practicing without distractions, asking your dog to sit or lie down, and rewarding them when they comply. Gradually introduce distractions such as knocking or ringing the doorbell while instructing them to maintain the sit or down position. Reward them for staying in place despite the excitement. Over time, and with consistency, your dog will learn to default to this behavior when they hear someone at the door.

Managing how your dog greets visitors involves preparation and cooperation from your guests. Inform visitors beforehand about what to expect and how they can help reinforce your dog's training. Ask them to ignore your dog upon entering if they start to jump.

Once your dog calmly sits or has all four paws on the ground, they can greet them with petting or treats. This helps reinforce the training and ensures that the behavior is consistently managed no matter who the visitor is. For dogs that struggle with over-excitement, having a unique set of toys or treats only used when guests arrive can help. These serve as a distraction and a reward for calm behavior, making the greetings process smoother and more enjoyable for everyone involved.

In your practice sessions, consider using a leash to control and guide your dog's movements when guests arrive. This added level of control can prevent jumping before it happens and reinforce the training in a safe, controlled manner. Remember, the goal isn't to punish the excitement but to channel it into acceptable behaviors that allow everyone to enjoy the interaction. As with any training, patience, consistency, and positive reinforcement are critical to success. With time and practice, your dog will learn that the best way to get attention and affection is not by jumping up but by keeping all four paws firmly on the ground.

DEALING WITH AGGRESSION: STRATEGIES FOR SAFETY AND IMPROVEMENT

Addressing aggression in dogs is a critical aspect of pet ownership, which requires understanding, patience, and sometimes professional intervention. Aggression can manifest in various forms and degrees, from growling and snapping to biting, and understanding the triggers—specific situations, people, or animals that provoke these responses—is essential in managing and eventually remedying this behavior.

The first step in addressing canine aggression is identifying what triggers your dog. These triggers can be as diverse as the presence of other dogs, discomfort with specific handling or grooming practices, territorial challenges, or fear-based reactions to unfamiliar people or situations. Keeping a detailed log of incidents can help you spot patterns and understand what environments or actions might contribute to your dog's aggression. For instance, if your dog only shows aggression during vet visits, the trigger might be fear of being restrained or pain. Alternatively, if aggression occurs only in the presence of other dogs, it could be rooted in poor socialization or past negative experiences with other dogs.

Once triggers are identified, implementing safety measures becomes paramount to prevent bites or fights. This might mean using a muzzle in public spaces or separating your dog in a safe room when visitors come over, depending on the severity and context of the aggression. Managing these situations carefully is crucial to avoid escalating aggression and protect your dog and others from harm. Additionally, simple changes in your daily routine and environment can decrease stress for your dog, reducing aggressive tendencies. For example, walking your dog during less busy times can prevent encounters with triggers, such as other dogs, that might lead to aggressive responses.

Behavior modification techniques are central to managing and eventually reducing aggression. These techniques often involve controlled exposure to the trigger and positive reinforcement to create new, positive associations. For example, if your dog is aggressive toward strangers, you might start by having a friend stand nearby where your dog notices them but doesn't react aggressively. You can then reward your dog for calm behavior with treats or praise. Gradually, as your dog becomes more comfortable, your friend can move closer, continuing to reinforce positive, non-aggressive behavior at each step. This technique, known as desensitization and counterconditioning, can be very effective but requires consistency and patience.

In cases where aggression is severe or poses a safety risk, seeking help from a professional is essential. An experienced dog trainer or a veterinary behaviorist can guide your situation. These professionals can help assess the underlying causes of aggression, develop a detailed behavior modification plan, and guide you through the training process. They can also determine whether medical factors might contribute to aggressive behavior and recommend medical therapies and behavioral training interventions.

Addressing aggression in dogs is not just about suppression or control; it's about understanding and managing the underlying causes. With the right strategies and support, most aggressive behaviors can be improved, leading to a safer and more harmonious relationship between you and your dog. Remember, the goal is not to punish your dog for their aggressive behavior but to help them feel secure and react more appropriately in situations that currently trigger their aggression. This approach enhances safety and contributes to your dog's overall well-being, helping them lead a happier and more balanced life.

OVERCOMING SEPARATION ANXIETY: A STEP-BY-STEP GUIDE

Separation anxiety in dogs is more than just a little whimpering when you grab your keys; it's a severe condition that can manifest in behaviors as mild as pacing and whining or as severe as destructive chewing and persistent howling. For many dogs, being alone triggers stress they can't manage independently. Understanding the signs and symptoms of this anxiety is your first step toward helping your beloved pet. Typically, these signs include excessive salivation, barking, scratching at doors or windows, attempting to escape from the house, and, in some cases, urinating or defecating inside when left alone. These behaviors are often misinterpreted as spiteful or naughty, but they're expressions of a deep-seated panic.

To address separation anxiety, start with gradual desensitization—essentially, get your dog used to being alone for short periods and slowly increase that time. Prepare to leave as usual, then step out momentarily before returning inside. It's essential to keep your departures and returns low-key to avoid creating a buzz around the act of leaving. Gradually extend the time you're gone by just a few minutes each session, and increase this time into hours over the coming weeks. Throughout this process, monitor your dog's behavior for signs of stress, and if they seem to be struggling, take a step back. This might mean reducing the time they're alone again until they're more comfortable.

Creating a safe space plays a pivotal role in this training. This space, whether a crate, a specific room, or a gated area, should feel like a sanctuary to your dog, filled with their favorite toys and comfort items like an old shirt that smells like you. The idea is to make this area so enjoyable and comforting that they voluntarily go there when they start their departure routine. The presence of familiar, comforting items can help ease their anxiety and make the space feel less like confinement and more like a safe retreat.

Addressing your dog's physical and mental needs is critical in easing separation anxiety. A well-experienced and mentally stimulated dog is less likely to feel anxious when left alone. This means regular exercise appropriate to your dog's age and health, such as walks, runs, or play sessions, should be a part of their daily routine. Engaging their mind with puzzle toys or treat-dispensing games can also help tire them out mentally. The goal is to leave your dog naturally tired and content, ideally ready for a nap, by the time you leave. This physical and mental exhaustion can make the alone time less stressful because they spend time sleeping and recuperating rather than fretting and feeling anxious.

Implementing these steps addresses the immediate behaviors associated with separation anxiety and helps build your dog's confidence in being alone. This confidence can lead to a more relaxed, happy pet that feels secure in its home environment, whether you are present or not. Remember, the key to success with these strategies is patience and consistency. Each dog will progress at its own pace, and understanding and responding to your dog's specific needs and reactions throughout this process will ultimately help them learn to cope with being alone.

LEASH REACTIVITY: TRAINING FOR CALM WALKS

Understanding leash reactivity is crucial for fostering pleasant and stress-free walks with your dog. It's important to note the difference between leash reactivity and aggression: *Leash reactivity* is generally triggered by being on a leash and feeling restricted, whereas *aggression* can occur in various situations and might involve more deliberate attempts to bite or attack. Leash reactivity, often mistaken for outright aggression, is typically a fear-based response to specific triggers when a dog feels restrained and unable to flee. Recognizing this behavior goes a long way toward managing it. Dogs may bark, lunge, or growl at other dogs, people, or vehicles, not necessarily out of aggression but often from anxiety or overexcitement. The triggers vary widely; some dogs react only to moving bikes, while others may respond to all passing animals or people. Observing your dog's behavior closely can help you identify the stimuli that trigger their reactivity.

Training for focus and control is pivotal in managing leash reactivity. Teaching your dog to maintain attention on you during walks can significantly mitigate reactive outbursts. Start with focus exercises in a quiet environment where your dog is less likely to be distracted. Use a cue like "look at me" or "watch," and reward them with treats or praise for maintaining eye contact. Gradually introduce more distractions as your dog becomes proficient at focusing on you in a calm setting. The goal is to build their ability to ignore distractions, no matter how tempting. Practice these exercises consistently, and over time, your dog will learn to look to you for cues on how to behave rather than instinctively reacting to their surroundings.

Counterconditioning is another effective strategy to change your dog's emotional response to the triggers of their reactivity. This technique involves associating the sight of a previous trigger with something positive, like their favorite treats or toys. For instance, if your dog reacts to other dogs on walks, begin by observing them from a distance, where your dog notices the other dog but does not react aggressively. At that moment, offer high-value treats or play a favorite game. Over time, and with repeated exposure, your dog will start associating the sight of other dogs with positive experiences, reducing their reactive behavior. This process requires patience and consistency, as changing deeply ingrained behaviors often takes time. It's also crucial to keep these training sessions short and positive, ending them before your dog becomes stressed or overwhelmed.

The choice of proper equipment can also impact the management of leash reactivity. While traditional collars can exacerbate the problem by increasing the feeling of restriction, specially designed no-pull harnesses can provide better control during walks without causing discomfort. These harnesses typically attach at the front of the chest, allowing you to steer your dog gently aside rather than pulling directly against their throat, which can provoke a more robust reactive response. The key is to choose a harness that fits well and does not restrict movement, ensuring that walks remain comfortable for your dog. Additionally, using a fixed-length leash rather than a retractable one gives you more control. It makes managing situations that might trigger their reactivity easier by preventing your dog from lunging forward unexpectedly.

You can transform your reactive dog's behavior on the leash by combining these strategies—understanding the triggers, training for focus and control, employing counterconditioning, and using appropriate walking equipment. The process requires understanding, patience, and dedication to consistent practice, resulting in a more relaxed and enjoyable walking experience for you and your dog. As you continue to work with your dog, remember that each small step forward is progress towards a calmer and happier shared path.

RESOURCE GUARDING: PREVENTION AND MANAGEMENT

Understanding why your dog may suddenly growl as you approach their food bowl or why they might snap when you reach for their favorite toy begins with recognizing the roots of resource guarding. This behavior is not about defiance or possessiveness as often perceived; it's an instinctual response rooted deeply in a dog's evolutionary history. In the wild, the ability to guard and protect valuable resources such as food, shelter, and mates was essential for survival. This natural tendency has persisted in domestic dogs, and while it may not be necessary for their survival now, it's a strong instinct that can manifest in various ways.

Resource guarding can vary in intensity—some dogs may only give a low growl or stiffen when someone approaches their food, while others might escalate to snapping or biting if they feel their prized possession is threatened. It's important to note that resource guarding is a normal dog behavior; however, in a family environment, it's crucial to manage it to ensure the safety and harmony of the household.

Prevention strategies are most effective when started in puppyhood but can also be adapted for adult dogs. The goal is to teach your dog that the human approach to their resource is a joyous event, not a threat. One effective method is to walk by and toss a tasty treat into their bowl while eating. This can help the dog associate your approach with good things rather than a potential loss. For toys, engage in trade games where you offer a treat or a more desirable toy in exchange for the one they have. This prevents guarding and teaches your dog polite ways to give up their resources.

The "trade" command is a helpful element in managing resource guarding. This involves teaching your dog to give up an item willingly in exchange for something better. Start with items that your dog values less, offering them a high-value treat in exchange for the item. Ensure the trade is always favorable to your dog, reinforcing that giving up something can lead to even better outcomes. You can gradually work with more valued items as your dog becomes more comfortable with this exchange. Stay consistent in this training to build a reliable response.

If resource guarding escalates or aggressive behaviors become apparent, consider professional intervention. Some resource guarding is severe and may pose a risk to family members, especially children who may not recognize the warning signs. Behaviorists and experienced trainers can provide targeted strategies that address your dog's needs, considering its history, environment, and family dynamics. These professionals are skilled in creating management and training plans that minimize risks and focus on modifying the guarding behavior, often using desensitization and counter-conditioning techniques tailored to your dog's specific triggers.

Resource guarding is a manageable behavior, but it requires understanding, patience, and consistent effort. By recognizing the signs early and implementing effective prevention and management strategies, you can help your dog learn to cope with their instincts in a manner that keeps everyone safe. The key is to foster an environment where your dog feels secure and is motivated to behave in ways that are compatible with your family life.

As we wrap up this chapter on common behavioral challenges, remember that each issue we've addressed, from barking to resource guarding, is rooted in natural canine behavior. Understanding and learning how to shape these instincts through training and management can enhance your relationship with your dog and contribute to a happier, more balanced home.

Looking ahead, we'll explore advanced training techniques that build on these foundations, offering ways to challenge and engage your dog further and strengthen the bond you share.

LEADING WITH THE BOND

There is nothing truer in this world than the love of a good dog.

— MIRA GRANT

As a dog owner and a lover of the species, it baffles me how many books lead with a focus on training. Of course, training is essential, and it's a massive part of how you create a special bond between you and your dog, but for me, the relationship comes first. That's *why* you want to train your dog: Keep them safe and nurture a bond with respectful boundaries and a genuine connection.

I guess you're inclined toward the same way of thinking – that's how you came to be reading this book – and you're likely to see far more success with your training because you focus on nurturing that bond and understanding your dog. I think this approach, when used more widely, would result in far more rewarding dog training experiences for both animals and their owners. I also know how unique the human-canine bond is; watching it unfold for others is a joy. This is why I wrote this book, and as someone with a similar way of looking at the world, you're the perfect person to help me spread this information to more people.

Tell your dog-owning friends about some of the nuggets you've discovered here, and tell them about this book. If you want to take it further and help me reach even more people and their four-legged friends, you can make a massive difference by leaving a review online.

By leaving a review of this book on Amazon, you'll show new readers where they can find all the information they need to

nurture a healthy and rewarding relationship with their dog.

Reviews connect readers with the books meant for them, and just a few words from you could make all the difference to someone's relationship with their dog.

Thank you so much for your support. The human-canine bond is something to be treasured, and I'm passionate about helping as many people as possible to nurture it.

SCAN ME

CHAPTER 5

ADVANCED TRAINING TECHNIQUES

O n a Thursday evening in Prescott, Arizona, a three-year-old girl was playing outside her home when she wandered into the vast desert. After several hours of searching for a ball, she realized she was lost. The family dog, Blue, a Queensland Heeler, was with her as she aimlessly ventured into the wilderness.

The next day, while searching for the girl, a Department of Public Safety helicopter crew observed ground movement where they spotted Blue circling the body of the child lying prone but alive in a creek bed three-quarters of a mile from her home. The Yavapai County Sheriff's Office spokesperson, Dwight D'Evelyn, credited Victoria Bensch's survival to her dog, Blue, who kept the child safe and warm when the overnight hours dropped to 30-degree temperatures. Victoria and the dog returned home and were reunited with her parents. The child was flown to Phoenix Children's Hospital, where she was treated for mild frostbite on her feet (The Arizona Republic, 2010).

A dog is an excellent playmate, companion, and guardian for children and adults. The loyalty and intelligence of the Queensland

Heeler are well-documented and admired. Society applauds when the media reports a good rescue dog story like Victoria's. Only then do we realize how necessary it could be to have our canine companion at our side.

My Queensland Heeler, Joey, is not just a pet but my constant companion. He trots alongside my bicycle when I ride it and prances at my side as we walk twice daily for hundreds, if not thousands, of miles over the years. His loyalty and endurance are unmatched. I consider us inseparable.

Joey is a natural source of security and comfort to me and my family. Victoria Bensch and I attest to this breed's unwavering watchfulness and devotion. The Queensland Heeler is proudly a cherished part of our lives.

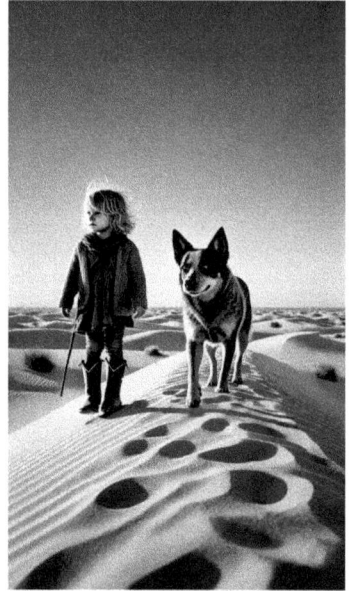

AGILITY TRAINING FOR FUN AND FITNESS

Imagine the sheer thrill of transforming your routine dog walks into an exhilarating blend of jumps, tunnels, and weave poles. That's the magic of agility training, a dynamic sport that turns ordinary exercises into exciting challenges for you and your dog. Agility training is a full-body workout that engages the mind, enhances coordination, and strengthens the bond between you and your canine companion. Visualize the joy on your dog's face as they zip through an obstacle course, their eyes sparkling with excitement and achievement—it's truly an exhilarating experience to witness.

Introduction to Agility

Agility training offers many benefits for both mental and physical health. For your dog, navigating through an agility course requires a combination of speed, flexibility, and problem-solving, which promotes mental alertness and physical fitness. The obstacles challenge them differently: Tunnels may encourage confidence, while weave poles foster nimble movements. For you, it's an opportunity to refine your communication skills and learn to give clear signals. Plus, it's quite the workout to keep up with your four-legged athlete! The beauty of agility lies in its adaptability; it can be as casual or competitive as you prefer, making it suitable for dogs (and owners) of all ages and fitness levels.

Getting Started with Agility

Embarking on agility training doesn't have to be complicated. You can start at home using everyday items to create simple obstacles. A broom balanced on two stacks of books can serve as a jump, while cones or rolled-up towels can be weaving poles. Introduce these obstacles gradually and ensure your dog's safety. Remember to shower your dog with encouragement and rewards to make the experience positive and enjoyable.

Joining a local club can also be a fantastic way to dive into agility training. Clubs often provide access to professional equipment and experienced trainers who can offer guidance tailored to your dog's level of expertise. However, clubs do not just offer training; you'll also find a sense of community and support there. Clubs are a great place to meet other dog owners who share your interest in agility training in a warm and welcoming environment where you can learn and grow together.

Building Confidence and Skill

As you and your dog master the basic agility tasks, the complexity and difficulty of the courses gradually increase. Start by chaining two obstacles together, then three, and so on. The key is to progress comfortably for your dog so they're confident and booming at each stage before moving on. This method helps incrementally build their confidence and skill, which is crucial for their development and enthusiasm for the sport.

Consistent practice, even just a few minutes daily, can enhance your dog's agility skills. It's not about lengthy, grueling sessions; agility should always be fun and rewarding. Keep sessions short and sweet, peppered with plenty of praise and treats. This approach ensures that agility training remains a delightful activity for your dog, keeping their motivation high.

Competition and Community

For those interested in exploring competitive agility, there are numerous options available. Local and national competitions provide a platform for you and your dog to test your skills against others, offering a structured environment where you can strive for excellence and recognition. Competing is about participating in a shared activity that deepens the connection between you and your dog, not just winning. The competitive environment also fosters a unique camaraderie among participants, who share tips, celebrate each other's successes, and enjoy the spirit of healthy competition.

Interactive Element: Agility Trial Journal

Consider keeping an agility trial journal. Document your training sessions, note improvements, and jot down areas needing work. This helps track your progress and is a reflective tool, allowing you to see how far you and your dog have come. After each competition or training session, take a moment to write down what went well and what could be improved. This habit can enhance your training strategy and provide a tangible record of your agility journey.

Agility training offers a delightful way to engage with your dog, providing physical and mental stimulation and a fantastic opportunity to strengthen your bond. Whether you choose to pursue it as a fun hobby or a competitive sport, agility training brings excitement and variety into your dog's life, ensuring they remain active, engaged, and happy.

SCENT WORK: ENGAGING YOUR DOG'S NATURAL ABILITIES

Imagine tapping into one of your dog's most powerful senses to enrich their life and boost their confidence. That's precisely what scent work accomplishes by leveraging your dog's natural sniffing abilities. Every dog has an incredible capacity to detect and differentiate scents, a skill honed over thousands of years. In the wild, this ability is crucial for finding food, detecting danger, and navigating the environment. Scent work as a training activity turns these instinctual behaviors into fun and mentally stimulating games that can deeply engage your dog, regardless of age, size, or breed.

The basics of scent work involve teaching your dog to identify and react to specific scents. You might begin with something simple, like a favorite treat or a familiar object, and hide it somewhere relatively easy for them to find. The goal is to challenge their nose and encourage them to use their brain to solve a puzzle. When your dog discovers the hidden scent, significant positive reinforcement—praise, a treat, or a favorite game—helps cement the connection between the task and the reward. This form of training taps into your dog's natural desire to hunt and track, providing a satisfying mental workout that is both enriching and exhausting, often more so than physical exercise alone. You'll feel a sense of accomplishment and pride when your dog successfully finds the hidden scent.

Setting up scent games at home can be simple, or you can get more creative. Start with a few cardboard boxes or open containers, each with holes large enough for the scent to escape but small enough to prevent your dog from seeing inside. Place a scented object in one of the boxes and encourage your dog to discover which holds the prize by using the command to "sniff it out" or "find it." As they become more adept at this game, you can increase the complexity by adding more boxes, using less potent scents, or creating a larger area for them to search. Another fun game involves scent trails. Using a cloth or a small brush, create a trail with the scent leading to a hidden object. This not only stimulates your dog's tracking ability but also adds an element of physical exercise to the mix.

You can introduce more complex scent work activities as your dog's skills improve. This might involve teaching them to identify specific scents beyond treats or familiar objects. Essential oils like lavender or vanilla are safe for dogs and can be used to create a scent discrimination game. Begin with one scented object among several unscented ones, gradually increasing the number of scented objects and the complexity of the task. Training your dog to participate in formal scent detection sports, like nose work competitions, can be an exciting challenge for those looking to take scent work further. These activities mimic professional detection dog tasks, requiring dogs to locate specific scents hidden in various environments.

The benefits of engaging in scent work extend beyond just having a good time. This training can improve your dog's focus as they learn to concentrate on a task despite distractions. It's also a fantastic confidence builder. Each successful find in a scent game provides a mental reward for your dog, reinforcing their problem-solving skills and boosting their confidence. Behaviorally, scent work can help calm anxious dogs by giving them a focused activity that occupies their mind and reduces stress. It's also inclusive—almost any dog can participate in scent work, making it a versatile activity for all kinds of dogs, from high-energy puppies to older dogs who might be less mobile but still mentally sharp.

By incorporating scent work into your regular interactive routines with your dog, you offer them a way to use their natural abilities in a fulfilling and enjoyable manner. This spices up their routine and deepens their bond as they work together to solve puzzles and explore new challenges. Whether laying a simple scent trail in your backyard or preparing for a competition, the world of scent work offers a fascinating way to see your dog's world, where their nose knows best.

TRICK TRAINING: STRENGTHENING BONDS THROUGH PLAYFUL LEARNING

Trick training is a delightful way to sprinkle magic into your routine, crafting moments that impress friends and family and deepen the bond between you and your furry friend. The key to successful trick training lies in selecting the right tricks that align with your dog's physical abilities, age, and size, ensuring that each new challenge perfectly fits their capabilities.

Choosing Tricks to Teach

Selecting the appropriate tricks is crucial and should be tailored to your dog's individual characteristics and health status. For a young, energetic puppy, tricks that involve a lot of movement, like "spin" or "jump through a hoop," can be ideal, as they burn off excess energy and keep them engaged. On the other hand, consider less physically demanding tricks such as "speak" or "shake hands" for older dogs or those with physical limitations. Always consider your dog's comfort and safety and avoid any tricks that might strain their joints or lead to injury. Observing your dog's reactions during initial attempts can also give valuable cues about their enjoyment and physical comfort with the trick.

Step-by-Step Training

Breaking down the training process into manageable steps is essential for effective learning. Let's take the trick "rollover" as an example. Start by having your dog in a "down" position. Then, hold a treat by their nose and slowly move it behind their shoulder, encouraging them to lie on their side. Continue guiding them with the treat so they complete a full roll. Throughout these steps, maintain a gentle and patient demeanor, ensuring each phase is clearly understood and mastered before moving on to the next. This gradual method helps build your dog's confidence and understanding, making the training session enjoyable and stress-free.

Positive Reinforcement

The backbone of successful trick training is positive reinforcement. This approach makes learning enjoyable and reinforces your dog's desire to please. The key is immediate and consistent reinforcement, which helps your dog associate the trick with positive outcomes. Whether it's treats, their favorite toy, or copious amounts of praise, ensure the reward is highly motivating and appropriate for the task. For instance, if the trick involves more extended activity, intersperse the training with play sessions to keep your dog excited and engaged. This keeps their energy levels up and turns the training session into a fun and rewarding game.

Creative and Fun Ideas

To keep trick training fresh and exciting, inject creativity into the tricks you choose to teach. Beyond the basic tricks like "sit" or "stay," explore unique and entertaining tricks such as "take a bow" or "play dead." These tricks add variety to your training sessions, stimulate your dog's cognitive abilities, and are great fun to showcase. You can also create tricks incorporating your dog's natural habits or behaviors, turning quirky behaviors into amusing and impressive ones. For example, if your dog naturally enjoys carrying objects, you might teach them to "fetch the newspaper" or "help with laundry" by picking up clothes. These tricks are entertaining and enhance your dog's ability to assist in everyday tasks, making them feel even more like an integral part of the family.

Incorporating these elements into your trick training sessions transforms them into a rich tapestry of interactive fun that benefits you and your dog. As you explore the vast array of tricks that your dog can master, remember that each small step they take is a leap towards greater confidence and a stronger bond between you both. Trick training is more than just teaching skills; it's about celebrating your unique connection with your canine companion through every shake, roll, and bow.

OFF-LEASH TRAINING: STEPS FOR SUCCESS

Imagine the freedom and joy your dog would experience, bounding through a park or along a trail, perfectly safe and under control with no leash to hold them back. This level of freedom can significantly enhance your dog's quality of life, but achieving it requires careful and thoughtful off-leash training. The foundation of successful off-leash training lies in a solid recall command. Recall, or the ability for your dog to come to you when called, is crucial. It ensures you can quickly regain control of your dog, preventing potential dangers from distractions or environmental hazards.

Start in a controlled environment with minimal distractions to build a reliable recall. Use a long-line leash for safety and give your dog a sense of freedom while maintaining control. Gradually increase the complexity of distractions as your dog's recall reliability improves. This training should be reinforced positively—treats, favorite toys, and enthusiastic praise can make returning to you the best part of your dog's playtime.

Safety is paramount when considering off-leash freedoms. Before you even unclip the leash, assess the environment for hazards such as nearby traffic, unfamiliar animals, or unsecured areas where your dog could get lost. It's also wise to ensure your dog is microchipped and wears a tag with your contact information, just in case they wander off. Initially, choose enclosed or semi-enclosed areas where your dog can explore without the risk of straying too far. Parks with designated off-leash areas designed with dogs in mind are safe options that provide both the freedom to explore and boundaries to keep your dog contained.

As they become more reliable in their recall and you grow more confident in their behavior, you can gradually introduce more open and challenging environments. Start by allowing them off-leash in secure, enclosed spaces to see how they respond to being untethered. Observe their willingness to stay close to you and their responsiveness to your commands. More training and a slower transition are necessary if they run off or become overly distracted. As they prove their reliability, you can gradually increase the freedom you allow them. This might mean transitioning from an enclosed park to a larger, open area. Throughout this process, continue practicing and reinforcing recall commands regularly, and always be prepared to step up the training again if your dog starts to regress or show less reliability.

Maintaining control and focus while off-leash is essential, especially in environments where distractions are plentiful. Training techniques that encourage your dog to check in with you regularly can be particularly effective. One method is the "ping-pong" technique, where you call your dog back to you, reward them, and then release them to play again. This reinforces the recall command and teaches your dog that checking in with you can be a rewarding experience. You can also use treats or toys to capture your dog's attention and bring them back to focus during off-leash outings. Always keep these sessions positive and full of energy, showing your dog that staying attentive to your commands is fun and rewarding.

Off-leash training allows your dog to explore the world freely and safely. It will enable your dog to satisfy its natural curiosities and exercise in a more engaging, fulfilling way. More importantly, it strengthens your trust and communication with your dog, reinforcing your bond and ensuring you enjoy off-leash adventures.

It would be best to remember that consistency is critical to building on these training foundations; practice and positive reinforcement help maintain the skills your dog has learned and ensure that they remain responsive and safe, no matter where your adventures take you.

BEHAVIORAL SHAPING: MODIFYING COMPLEX BEHAVIORS

Shaping complex behaviors in dogs through successive approximations is akin to sculpting a masterpiece from a rough block of marble. Each small chisel, each subtle refinement, gradually reveals the form hidden within. In dog training, shaping involves breaking down a desired complex behavior into smaller, manageable components, rewarding your dog at each incremental step until the entire behavior is achieved. This method harnesses the power of positive reinforcement to mold behaviors over time, making it an effective technique for teaching intricate tasks that your dog may not naturally perform.

The concept of shaping can be applied to various behaviors, from simple tricks like ringing a bell to go outside to more complex behaviors like assisting with household chores. For instance, if you want to teach your dog to fetch the newspaper, you would start by rewarding them for approaching the newspaper, then for touching it, and gradually for picking it up, carrying it, and finally bringing it to you. Each step builds upon the previous one, using positive reinforcements such as treats or praises to encourage your dog and reinforce the behavior at each stage. This method makes learning more digestible for your dog and turns training into a fun and rewarding activity, enhancing your bond.

Creating a Shaping Plan

Developing a successful shaping plan for your dog involves careful observation, patience, and a systematic approach. Start by clearly defining the end behavior you want to teach. Once you have a clear goal, brainstorm the steps your dog will need to take to reach that goal, breaking the behavior down into the smallest possible increments. These steps should be simple enough for your dog to achieve relatively quickly, ensuring that each action can be identified and rewarded.

Next, consider the best way to motivate your dog. Each dog is unique, and what works for one might not work for another. Some dogs may be highly food-motivated, while others might respond better to toys or verbal praise. Select a desirable and appropriate reward for the task and be ready to offer it immediately after your dog performs the desired behavior. This immediacy helps your dog make a clear association between the action and the reward, reinforcing the behavior more effectively.

As you begin training, please start with the first, most straightforward behavior and move on to the next step once your dog performs it consistently and reliably. This might require several training sessions, and that's okay. Shaping is about accuracy and building confidence. If your dog seems confused or frustrated, it may be necessary to break the steps down even further or spend more time reinforcing earlier steps—successful shaping results from flexibility in your plan and responding to your dog's needs.

Examples of Successful Shaping

Real-life success stories abound in behavioral shaping, demonstrating its effectiveness and versatility. Take, for instance, a service dog named Bella, trained to assist her owner, who uses a wheelchair. Bella's training included learning to open doors, a complex behavior shaped over several months. Initially, Bella was rewarded simply for touching a tug rope attached to the door handle. Gradually, the behavior was shaped to include pulling on the rope, moving the door slightly, and finally opening it wide enough for her owner to pass through. Each step was carefully planned and positively reinforced, leading to a successful outcome that improved her owner's quality of life.

Another example involves a rescue dog named Max, who initially feared human contact. Through shaping, Max was gradually desensitized to human interaction, starting with being rewarded for calmly observing a person from a distance, allowing a person to approach him, and eventually initiating contact. This careful, step-by-step approach helped Max overcome his fears and develop trust in people, transforming him from a skittish stray into a loving, affectionate companion.

These stories highlight the transformative power of behavioral shaping, illustrating how it can teach new skills, modify existing behaviors, and overcome challenges. Whether you're looking to teach your dog a new trick, have them assist with disabilities, or modify problematic behaviors, shaping offers a flexible, practical, and advantageous approach to achieving your training goals.

THERAPY AND SERVICE DOG BASICS: TRAINING FOR A PURPOSE

When you think of dogs that work, two distinct types often come to mind: therapy and service dogs. Both play invaluable roles in assisting humans, yet their responsibilities, training, and the laws that protect them differ significantly. Anyone who considers training their dog in one of these capacities or learning more about these remarkable animals needs to understand the distinction between the two.

Therapy dogs are trained to provide comfort and affection to individuals in hospitals, nursing homes, schools, and other settings. They are not trained to perform specific tasks for individuals with disabilities; they offer emotional support to various people they meet in therapeutic or educational environments. Service dogs, on the other hand, are trained to perform specific tasks that assist individuals with disabilities, such as guiding people who are blind, alerting individuals who are deaf, pulling a wheelchair, or even reminding a person to take prescribed medications. Consequently, the training for service dogs is more rigorous and tailored to the specific needs of the handler.

The foundational skills for therapy and service dogs include basic obedience such as sit, stay, come, down, and heel. Beyond these basics, the training diverges significantly. Therapy dogs must be adaptable, friendly, comfortable in various environments, and exhibit an innate calmness and affection towards strangers. Service dogs, meanwhile, require a higher level of discipline and must be able to perform specific tasks reliably in all environments. A key temperament trait for both is a calm disposition; however, service dogs must also have a high focus and independence to effectively assist their handler with specific needs.

Training a therapy or service dog involves not just the handler and the dog but often professional trainers as well. Both dogs' certification processes ensure they meet health, safety, and training standards. Therapy dogs typically undergo evaluations that test their behavior in various social situations, handling of unfamiliar noises and equipment, and reactions to different types of people. Service dogs, however, must pass similar assessments and demonstrate their ability to perform the specific tasks for which they have been trained. In the United States, the Americans with Disabilities Act (ADA) provides legal protection for service dogs, allowing them access to all public spaces when accompanying their handlers. Therapy dogs do not receive the same legal protections and are generally only allowed onto public or private properties by invitation or arrangement.

Therapy and service dogs have a deep impact on individuals and communities. Therapy dogs have been shown to reduce stress, increase patient responsiveness, and improve the overall atmosphere in medical and educational facilities. Service dogs offer their handlers increased independence, safety, and improved mental health. The presence of a service dog can decrease the need for human caretakers and provide a sense of security and companionship for individuals with disabilities.

These dogs do more than help; they transform lives, offering independence, safety, and emotional support in unique and powerful ways. As you consider the role of working dogs in society, remember that their impact goes beyond their tasks. They are not just pets or helpers but critical contributors to the well-being and independence of many individuals, offering not only assistance but also companionship and unconditional love.

As this chapter closes, reflect on the remarkable abilities of these dogs and the training that empowers them to change lives. This section has highlighted not only the skills necessary for therapy and service dogs but also their mighty impact on individuals and communities, enhancing our understanding of the capabilities and contributions of these extraordinary animals.

CHAPTER 6

THE HEALTHY DOG

❧

I magine a day filled with your dog's vibrant energy and joyful antics, where their every action seems to spring from a well of endless vitality. Now, consider how different that day might look if your dog were lazy, uninterested, or irritable. It's not something any dog owner wants to think about. Still, the reality is that much of your dog's energy and behavior stem from something surprisingly simple and entirely within your control: their diet.

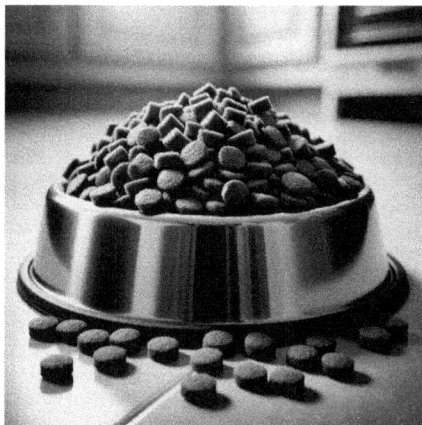

NUTRITION'S ROLE IN BEHAVIOR

Diet and Behavior Connection

There is an undeniable link between what your dog eats and how they feel and behave. Nutrition impacts your dog's energy levels, mood, and overall behavior. A well-balanced diet can lead to a well-balanced dog who exhibits fewer behavioral problems such as excessive barking, anxiety, or aggression. Conversely, a diet lacking essential nutrients may contribute to noticeable declines in energy and mood and even exacerbate or lead to behavioral issues. For instance, diets high in carbohydrates can cause spikes and crashes in blood sugar levels, which may contribute to hyperactivity, followed by lethargy. Insufficient protein can lead to a lack of amino acids like tryptophan, which is critical for producing serotonin. This hormone helps regulate mood and anxiety in humans and dogs.

Understanding these connections can empower you to make informed choices about your dog's diet, which can have a tangible impact on daily behavior and long-term health. The quality and composition of your dog's diet matter as much as the amount of food your dog eats.

Choosing the Right Diet

Given the many options available, selecting the proper diet for your dog can seem daunting. Still, it boils down to understanding your dog's specific needs, which can vary based on their age, breed, activity level, and any health issues they might have. The goal is to provide a balanced diet that meets all their nutritional requirements. High-quality commercial dog foods usually offer complete nutrition, and they often come in formulations targeted at specific life stages or health needs, such as puppy growth, weight management, or senior dog care. However, it's always a good idea to read ingredient labels and choose a diet that lists real meat as one of the top ingredients, ensuring your dog gets a high-quality protein source.

If commercial diets don't seem to suit your dog, or if you prefer a more hands-on approach, home-cooked meals or a raw diet are options that can offer personalized nutrition tailored to your dog's individual preferences and health requirements but require more effort and careful planning. A veterinarian or a pet nutritionist can provide valuable guidance when designing a diet plan that ensures your dog gets the necessary nutrients in the correct proportions.

Supplements and Behavior

Supplements can be critical in addressing specific behavioral issues linked to nutritional deficiencies. For example, omega-3 fatty acids, commonly found in fish oils, are known for their anti-inflammatory effects and can also aid in brain function, potentially reducing anxiety and improving mood. Probiotics are another supplement that can influence behavior by promoting a healthy gut, and they are linked to producing neurotransmitters that affect mood and behavior.

When considering supplements, consult your veterinarian, who can recommend safe and effective products. Also, remember that supplements should complement, not replace, a well-balanced diet.

Common Dietary Triggers

Some foods can enhance your dog's behavior and mood, but others can trigger adverse reactions. Common dietary triggers include excessive amounts of artificial additives, such as colors and preservatives, which some studies suggest may lead to hyperactivity and other behavioral changes. Gluten and excessive grain fillers can also cause issues, especially for dogs with sensitivities or allergies. These can manifest physically and through changes in behavior, such as increased irritability or anxiety.

Being aware of these triggers and understanding how to identify them on food labels can help you avoid selecting foods that might negatively impact your dog's behavior. Conducting an elimination diet under veterinary supervision can help pinpoint specific ingredients to which your dog might react.

Interactive Element: Dietary Journal

Consider keeping a dietary journal for your dog. This can be a simple notebook where you record what your dog eats, how much, and their behavior after each meal. Over time, this journal can provide insights into how different foods affect your dog, helping you make more informed dietary choices that enhance their well-being and behavior.

Incorporating thoughtful, informed choices about your dog's nutrition allows you to nourish their whole being—body and mind. As you continue to explore the impact of diet on your dog's behavior, remember that each meal is an opportunity to positively influence their health, happiness, and quality of life.

THE IMPACT OF EXERCISE ON MENTAL HEALTH

When you toss a ball across the yard or watch your dog sprint with unbridled joy, you're doing more than giving them a physical workout; you're contributing to their mental well-being. The impact of regular exercise on a dog's mental health is profound and multifaceted, influencing everything from their mood to their behavior. Just as humans feel a sense of calm after a good workout, dogs reap the emotional benefits of physical activity, which can be a powerful tool in managing anxiety, aggression, and other behavioral issues like chewing on the couch or escaping through an open door.

Exercise Requirements

Your dog's exercise needs can vary widely depending on their breed, age, and health. For instance, young, energetic breeds like Border Collies or Labrador Retrievers typically require more vigorous and frequent exercise to satisfy their innate energy levels. Without adequate physical activity, these dogs can develop destructive behaviors to expel unused energy. On the other hand, older dogs or breeds with lower energy levels, such as Bulldogs or older Basset Hounds, might require less intense activities to keep them. Tailoring your dog's exercise routine to their specific needs is essential to ensure they get enough activity to stay healthy without risking injury or exhaustion.

Regular exercise not only keeps your dog physically fit but also aids in maintaining their mental health. It helps mitigate symptoms of anxiety and depression by releasing endorphins, the body's natural stress relievers. For dogs with tendencies toward aggression or hyperactivity, regular physical activity is an outlet to expend excess energy and reduces the likelihood of such behaviors manifesting. It's a simple equation: A tired dog is typically happy and more relaxed.

Behavioral Benefits of Exercise

The behavioral benefits of regular exercise are particularly noticeable in dogs with anxiety issues. Activities that burn off energy can help lessen the intensity of anxiety-related behaviors like excessive barking or chewing. Exercise also helps establish a routine, providing a comforting structure for anxious pets and making the world seem more predictable and less threatening. For dogs that display signs of aggression, engaging them in regular exercise can reduce the frequency and intensity of these behaviors. Physical activity helps them manage their emotions better and makes them less likely to react aggressively under stress.

Creative Exercise Options

While walks and games of fetch are great, there are other ways to keep your dog engaged physically and mentally. Consider activities that challenge their mind as well as their body. Agility training, for instance, is not only a fantastic physical exercise but also requires them to think about and anticipate obstacles, which keeps their brain active and engaged. Puzzle toys that release treats as they are solved can be another excellent way to keep your dog's body and mind active, especially on days when long outdoor activities might not be possible.

Another fun option is setting up a DIY obstacle course using household items or inexpensive agility equipment in your backyard or living room. This provides physical exercise and strengthens your bond with your dog as you work through the course together. For those with access to safe water bodies, swimming can be an excellent exercise for dogs, especially for those with joint issues, as it is low impact yet highly effective in burning energy.

Monitoring Exercise

While exercise is beneficial, owners must ensure it is done within safe limits. Monitoring your dog during physical activities is essential so they do not overexert themselves, especially in hot weather when the risk of heatstroke is higher. Signs of overexertion include excessive panting, drooling, lethargy, or even collapse. Always allow your dog access to fresh water, and try to exercise during cooler parts of the day during hot weather. After exercise, observe your dog for any signs of discomfort or pain, which could indicate that the activity was too strenuous.

Regular vet checkups can help assess whether your dog's exercise routine is appropriate for its health status. Make adjustments based on professional advice. Considering these factors, you can create a balanced exercise regimen that keeps your dog physically fit and mentally sharp, enriching its quality of life.

RECOGNIZING AND ADDRESSING PAIN IN DOGS

When your dog starts to act out-of-sorts, it's not always easy to tell what might be wrong. Unlike humans, dogs can't verbally tell us when they're in pain, so it falls on us, their caretakers, to read their signs and signals. Recognizing when your dog is in pain is the first step towards helping them feel better. The signs can be subtle or obvious, ranging from physical manifestations to changes in behavior. Physically, a dog in pain might limp, have difficulty getting up or lying down, show decreased activity, or react negatively to being touched in certain areas. Behaviorally, they might exhibit increased vocalization like whimpering or growling or show signs of agitation and restlessness. Changes in their eating and sleeping habits or a sudden shift in their interaction with other pets and family members can also indicate discomfort.

Understanding these signs is vital because pain can significantly alter a dog's quality of life. It can affect their ability to enjoy regular activities, lead to behavioral changes, and, if left unaddressed, can evolve into more severe health issues. Once you suspect your dog might be in pain, consult your veterinarian. They can help determine the cause of the pain and recommend appropriate treatment options. Pain management might include medications such as anti-inflammatories, physical therapy, or, in some cases, more advanced treatments like acupuncture or surgery, depending on the underlying cause. Home care also plays an important role in managing your dog's pain. This can involve providing a comfortable resting area or making slight adjustments in their diet.

Impact of Pain on Behavior

Pain doesn't just affect your dog's physical health; it impacts their behavior. Dogs in pain may exhibit increased aggression, anxiety, or withdrawal, behaviors that are often misunderstood as lousy behavior rather than expressions of discomfort. For instance, a usually friendly dog might start to snap or growl when approached or touched, which can be misinterpreted as aggression. However, this is often their way of communicating discomfort and protecting themselves from further pain. Recognizing that these behavioral changes are symptoms of pain can help prevent misunderstandings and ensure your dog receives the necessary care. Addressing the root cause of the pain is crucial to alleviating their physical discomfort and helping them return to their standard behavioral patterns. Without proper treatment, pain can lead to a decline in mental health, affecting their overall well-being and potentially leading to more serious behavioral issues.

Preventative Measures

Prevention is always better than cure, and this is particularly true when it comes to managing your dog's health. One of the best ways to prevent injuries and conditions leading to chronic pain is by exercising regularly and maintaining a healthy weight. Obesity in dogs can lead to joint pain and other health issues that can impact their quality of life. Ensuring your dog gets appropriate exercise tailored to their breed, age, and health status can help maintain their physical health and prevent the onset of pain-related conditions. Additionally, regular vet checkups are essential. These mitigate any emerging health issues that could lead to pain and provide an opportunity to discuss and update pain prevention strategies tailored to your dog's needs.

Another aspect of prevention is being mindful of your dog's environment. For example, ensuring that your home is safe and free from hazards that could cause injury, such as slippery floors or unsafe stairs, is crucial. Simple modifications like ramps or steps to help aging dogs get on and off higher surfaces can prevent painful injuries. Regular grooming and nail trims can also prevent overgrown nails, which can lead to pain and difficulty walking.

Understanding and preventing pain in your dog involves vigilance, regular health care, and environmental management. By staying attuned to your dog's needs and behaviors, ensuring they remain physically active and healthy, and making necessary adjustments to their living conditions, you can help safeguard their well-being and prevent pain from diminishing the quality of life they deserve.

THE IMPORTANCE OF REGULAR VETERINARY CHECKUPS

Regular veterinary checkups ensure your furry companion's health and happiness. Think of these visits not just as routine examinations but as preventive measures to safeguard your dog from numerous health issues that could go unnoticed. Like humans, dogs can develop health conditions that aren't immediately obvious. Regular checkups help catch these before they become serious, ensuring your dog remains healthy and vibrant. For instance, early detection of conditions like heart disease or diabetes can make a difference in management options and outcomes. Vets can run various tests during these checkups to monitor your dog's health, including blood tests, urinalysis, and parasitic screenings, which can reveal hidden problems that are not evident through a physical examination alone.

Beyond physical health, veterinarians also play a crucial role in addressing and managing behavioral issues. This is especially important because sometimes, changes in behavior are the first signs of health problems. For example, if your once energetic dog suddenly seems lethargic or uninterested in activities they used to enjoy, this could be a sign of underlying issues such as thyroid problems or arthritis. During a checkup, you can discuss these behavioral changes, and your vet can advise whether they warrant further investigation or treatment. In cases where the behavior may be linked to psychological factors like anxiety or stress, veterinarians can provide initial guidance and, if necessary, refer you to a veterinary behaviorist who specializes in deeper behavioral issues. This holistic approach addresses your dog's physical and mental health needs.

Regarding preventive care, Staying up to date with vaccinations is vital to protect your dog from various infectious diseases that affect dogs of all ages. Your vet can guide you on which vaccinations are necessary and when they should be administered based on your dog's age, lifestyle, and the prevalent health risks in your area. Preventative treatments also extend to regular deworming and flea and tick control, which protect your dog and help maintain a safe and healthy environment for everyone in the home.

Building a positive and communicative relationship with your veterinarian is another fundamental aspect of your dog's health care. Start by ensuring that every visit to the vet is as stress-free as possible. You can do this by acclimatizing your dog to the car rides and the vet's office environment from a young age. Treats, positive reinforcement, and calm behavior can help make vet visits a more pleasant experience for your dog. Always be open and honest with your vet about any observations or concerns you have about your dog's health or behavior. A good vet will appreciate your insights and consider them valuable in assessing your dog's health.

Remember, you know your dog best; your observations can provide crucial context for diagnostics.

Integrating Journaling into Vet Visits

Consider keeping a health journal for your dog to take along to your vet visits. Record any symptoms, behavioral changes, eating habits, and even your dog's reactions to new diets or environments. This journal can give your vet a comprehensive view of your dog's health over time, making it easier to spot trends or changes that might indicate health issues. This proactive approach can make all the difference in managing your dog's health, ensuring they lead a long, happy, and healthy life.

By embracing these practices, you actively contribute to the well-being of your beloved pet. Regular vet checkups, vigilance, and commitment to following professional advice are the cornerstone of effective preventive health care. Remember, these visits are more than just a routine formality; they are integral to catching health issues early, understanding and managing behavioral concerns, and ensuring your dog's vaccinations and treatments are updated. Together with your vet, you are partners in maintaining the health and happiness of your dog.

INTEGRATING MENTAL STIMULATION INTO DAILY ROUTINES

Mental stimulation for dogs, often referred to as "brain games," plays a pivotal role in their overall well-being, akin to the effect mental exercise has on human health. Just as humans require intellectual challenges to stay sharp and ward off boredom, our canine companions thrive when their days involve more than basic physical activities and rest. Mental enrichment can prevent a range of undesirable behaviors that stem from boredom and lack of stimulation, such as destructive chewing, incessant barking, or even anxiety. Engaging your dog's brain daily helps to keep them mentally sharp, emotionally balanced, and deeply connected to you as their caregiver and guide through life's adventures.

Incorporating mental stimulation into your dog's routine can be straightforward. It can be as simple as turning meal times into a puzzle or as elaborate as teaching new tricks and skills. For instance, instead of feeding your dog from a bowl, use a puzzle feeder or scatter their kibble in the yard or around the house, encouraging them to use their problem-solving skills and sense of smell to find their food. This slows their eating, which is better for their digestion and provides a fun challenge that keeps boredom at bay.

Another simple yet effective way to integrate mental stimulation into daily routines is through "hide and seek" games, either with treats or with yourself. Hiding treats around your home or hiding and calling your dog to come and find you can be a thrilling and rewarding game that utilizes their natural sniffing and tracking abilities. These activities encourage your dog to think and solve problems, which enhances their cognitive faculties and provides a satisfying mental workout.

DIY Enrichment Toys

For those who enjoy crafting and DIY projects, creating homemade toys and games can be a fun and cost-effective way to stimulate your dog mentally. A straightforward project is a homemade snuffle mat. These mats are made from fleece or old fabric tied onto a rubber mat with holes, and they become a soft, dense forest of fabric strips where you can hide kibble or treats. As your dog snuffles through the mat, it engages its brain and senses to hunt for hidden treasures, providing mental and olfactory stimulation.

Another DIY project involves creating a puzzle box. Fill a small cardboard box with safe, non-toxic items like balled-up paper or old toilet rolls. Hide treats within this setup and seal the box lightly so your dog can rip it open to access the rewards. This stimulates your dog's brain and satisfies its natural shredding instincts in a controlled and safe environment. Always supervise your dog with DIY toys to ensure they do not ingest non-edible materials.

Recognizing Signs of Boredom

Knowing when your dog needs more mental engagement is crucial in maintaining health. Signs of boredom can sometimes be subtle but often include pacing, whining, or showing an unusual interest in things they usually ignore, like the walls or furniture. More obvious signs include destructive behavior or attempts to escape from the house or yard. These behaviors are your dog's way of trying to find something stimulating to do, and they often occur when their environment lacks sufficient mental challenges.

Effectively addressing boredom means assessing and adjusting your dog's daily activities to include more engaging, mentally stimulating tasks. It's important to balance physical exercise, training, play, and mental challenges that cater to your dog's specific needs and natural tendencies. Each dog is unique, and what works for one may not work for another, so it's essential to experiment with different activities and toys to discover what keeps your dog engaged and happy.

Integrating these practices into your routine gives your dog the physical activity and mental stimulation they need for their well-being. This holistic approach to pet care helps your dog remain physically fit and mentally sharp, fostering a content, vibrant life and a deep, fulfilling bond between you.

THE BENEFITS OF ROUTINE AND STRUCTURE

Creating a stable and predictable environment for your dog can improve their behavior and overall well-being. Just as humans benefit from a regular schedule, dogs, too, thrive on routine. A consistent daily schedule helps reduce stress and anxiety in dogs by providing a predictable environment. This predictability helps them feel secure so they know what to expect next, which can decrease behaviors borne out of anxiety, such as excessive barking, chewing, or even aggression. Setting times for meals, walks, play, and rest helps regulate your dog's internal clock and makes them calmer and more content.

The structure isn't just about sticking to a timetable; it's about creating a balance that meets all your dog's needs. For instance, morning might be the best time for a brisk walk when your dog is full of energy, followed by some training exercises to engage their mind. Interactive play can come later in the day, which helps strengthen your bond and provides essential social interaction. Scheduled downtimes, such as after meals or in the late evening, provide necessary rest and digestion periods. This balanced schedule keeps your dog physically active and mentally sharp and helps prevent overstimulation and fatigue, which can lead to irritability or hyperactivity.

As your dog grows and transitions through different stages of life, their needs will inevitably change, and so will their routine. Puppies, for instance, require more sleep and frequent but shorter bursts of exercise and training to accommodate their developing bodies and attention spans. On the other hand, senior dogs might need more rest periods and less intense activities to suit their aging bodies. Health issues might also necessitate adjustments in their routine—for example, a dog recovering from surgery may need more time indoors and limited physical activity. Their behavior will often be the first indicator that a change is needed; perhaps they are less enthusiastic about long walks or are sleeping more than usual. Listening to and observing your dog will be vital in making these adjustments.

The Role of Structure in Training

Incorporating structure into your training sessions can enhance their effectiveness. Structured training involves setting clear goals for each session, using consistent commands, and maintaining a routine that gradually builds on previously learned skills. This consistency helps reinforce learning and makes the training process smoother and more successful. For example, if you teach your dog to sit, consistently using the same command in a designated training spot can help your dog understand and respond quickly. Similarly, ending each session with a particular signal or command can help them know that training is over, which can prevent confusion and help them transition back to other activities more comfortably.

This predictability not only aids in learning but also strengthens the human-canine bond. Dogs are naturally inclined to look to their owners for cues on behavior. A structured approach to training and daily life helps build trust and respect, showing your dog you are reliable and consistent. Over time, this can make your dog more responsive to you, fostering a deeper connection and understanding between you.

Integrating these routine and structure elements into daily interactions with your dog creates a nurturing environment that promotes good behavior and a strong, loving relationship. This approach lays a solid foundation for a happy, well-adjusted dog who is a joy to be around and feels secure and valued in their family unit.

As we wrap up this chapter on establishing routine and structure in your dog's life, we've explored how a predictable environment can enhance your dog's behavioral health, the importance of creating a balanced schedule, and the necessity of adjusting routines to match your dog's evolving needs. We also explored how structured interactions, particularly in training, can bolster the effectiveness of your efforts and deepen the bond you share with your canine companion.

Moving forward, the insights and strategies discussed here serve as a foundation that supports not just your dog's physical and behavioral health but also the emotional and psychological well-being that makes them such cherished members of our families. As we continue into the next chapter, we will build on these principles, exploring more advanced techniques and ideas for enriching your life with your dog. This journey is not just about training or routine —it's about enriching the connection you share with your loyal companion.

CHAPTER 7

REAL-LIFE SUCCESS STORIES

E very dog has a story, and sometimes, these stories transcend the ordinary, teaching us lessons about resilience, adaptation, and the transformative power of love and patience. This chapter delves into the heartwarming narrative of a rescue dog whose journey from aggression to affection illustrates the remarkable impact of compassionate training and understanding.

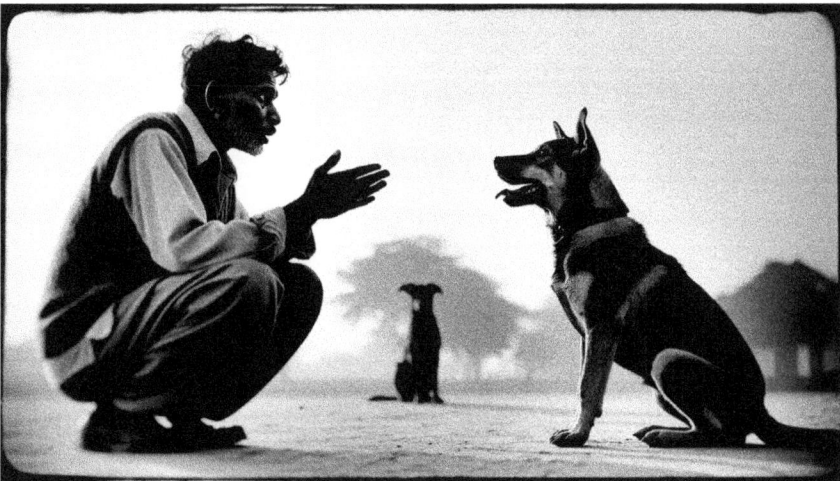

FROM AGGRESSIVE TO AFFECTIONATE: A RESCUE DOG'S JOURNEY

Understanding the Roots of Aggression

Imagine adopting a dog whose past is a mystery and whose first instinct is to snap and growl when approached. This was the case with my dog Koa Bear, a large-sized Akbash livestock guardian dog with a history of neglect and possible abuse. Koa's aggressive behaviors were deeply rooted in his past experiences, where his world was likely one of survival and mistrust. For many dogs like Koa, aggression is often not a trait but a learned behavior stemming from fear, insecurity, or traumatic experiences. Understanding this was the first step in helping Koa transform from a fearful aggressor to a loving companion.

The Power of Positive Reinforcement

The journey began with positive reinforcement training, which focuses on rewarding desired behaviors and encouraging the dog to repeat them. For Koa, whose previous encounters with humans might have involved punishment or harsh treatment, experiencing positive reinforcement was both novel and challenging. We started with simple commands that could be achieved easily and rewarded heavily. Each time Koa responded to a command without aggression, he was rewarded with his favorite treats and lots of praise. Slowly, he began associating human interactions with positive outcomes, reshaping his expectations and reactions.

Building Trust and Confidence

Building trust with Koa Bear was like carefully constructing a bridge over a chasm of doubt and fear. Every small step Koa took towards trusting humans was met with consistent, gentle encouragement. We introduced new people gradually, ensuring these interactions were controlled and positive. Over time, Koa has learned to greet strangers without fear or aggression. This growing trust significantly altered his demeanor, replacing his anxiety and aggression with curiosity and a desire for affection. His confidence blossomed, showing how much potential lay beneath his once-guarded exterior.

Celebrating Milestones

Each milestone in Koa's journey was celebrated as a monumental success. Every moment was acknowledged, from the first day he allowed a stranger to pet him without showing aggression to the joyful abandon with which he eventually played with other dogs. These celebrations were crucial for Koa Bear and those involved in his rehabilitation. They served as reminders of the deep changes that were taking place, fueling our commitment to his journey.

Interactive Element: Reflective Journaling Prompt

Consider keeping a journal of your dog's training progress, similar to Koa Bear's story. Record the challenges faced, the strategies implemented, and the successes achieved, no matter how small. This reflective practice allows you to track your dog's progress and serves as a motivational tool, reminding you of the journey taken and the transformations achieved. Here's a prompt to get you started: Reflect on a moment when your dog surprised you with their progress. What emotions did you feel, and what did this moment teach you about your dog's capabilities?

As we continue to explore more stories in this chapter, Koa's life stands as a testament to the inherent potential in every dog, waiting to be unlocked through patience, understanding, and the right approach to training. Each story highlights individual triumphs and underscores the universal themes of trust, transformation, and the incredible bond that can develop between dogs and humans.

THE SENIOR DOG WHO LEARNED NEW TRICKS

It's a common misconception that you can't teach an old dog a new trick, but time and again, senior dogs like Joey prove this adage wrong. Joey, a brightly spotted Cattle Dog of twelve years, came into my life with a gentle demeanor and the slow pace typical of older dogs. Many believe that once a dog reaches a certain age, their capacity for learning wanes, their curiosity dims, and their world narrows. However, the truth is that senior dogs have an incredible capacity to adapt and learn; it just requires a shift in our approach and expectations.

Training older dogs like Joey requires patience, understanding, and adaptability. Unlike younger dogs, seniors might have limitations such as reduced hearing, sight, or mobility, and their cognitive processing might be slower. It's crucial, therefore, to tailor training sessions to accommodate these changes. For Joey, this meant shorter training sessions to match his shorter attention span and incorporating more tactile cues to compensate for his diminished hearing. The focus was always on making each session enjoyable and stress-free, using plenty of positive reinforcements such as soft verbal praise and his favorite treats, which were small and easy on his older teeth.

Teaching Joey new tricks was not just about keeping him physically engaged but also beneficial for his mental health. Each new trick I taught Joey was a small victory against the encroaching isolation often accompanying an aging dog's life. Learning to "shake hands," "roll over," or even "play dead" gave Joey physical stimulation and mental challenges that kept his mind sharp. These activities helped mitigate the typical age-related decline in cognitive function, keeping his neurons firing and synapses active. Moreover, his joy and excitement with each successful trick were clear indicators of his thriving spirit, showing how such mental exercises could enhance his quality of life.

However, the most beautiful aspect of teaching Joey new tricks was the deepening of our bond. Each training session allowed us to connect, communicate, and understand each other better. This shared activity strengthened our trust and affection, proving that the emotional connections we forge with our dogs do not diminish with age; they can grow even more vital. Witnessing Joey's glee as he mastered a new trick or his eager anticipation at the start of each session was a poignant reminder of the enduring capacity for joy and engagement in senior dogs.

Success Story: Joey's New Chapter

Joey's journey into learning as a senior dog was not just about the tricks. When he arrived, Joey seemed to have accepted a quieter, more sedate lifestyle. However, as we progressed in our training, there was a visible shift in his demeanor. He became more engaged and connected, not just with me but with everyone around him. His eyes sparkled with an infectious vivacity, and his tail wagged with a vigor that belied his years.

One of Joey's standout moments came during a family gathering when he proudly demonstrated his new tricks. The delight and surprise on the faces of family members, as Joey performed his "play dead" trick, were unforgettable. For us, it wasn't just about the trick but about challenging and changing people's perceptions of what an older dog can achieve. Joey wasn't just learning new tricks; he was teaching us all a valuable lesson about resilience, capability, and the often-untapped potential of senior dogs.

Joey's story is a testament to the fact that age is not a barrier to learning or living a vibrant life. It's a reminder that our senior dogs have much to offer, and they can teach us if we provide them with the opportunities and support they need. Each senior dog, like Joey, has the potential to start a new chapter, one filled with learning, growth, and an abundance of joy, proving that, indeed, you can teach an old dog a new trick, and sometimes, they might teach us a few lessons in return.

THE ANXIOUS DOG WHO FOUND CALM

In the tapestry of canine behaviors, anxiety can manifest as a subtle thread that gradually weaves its way through a dog's actions and interactions. For Hapa, a fisty-tempered Mini-Australian Shepherd with a shadow of anxiety following her every move, the journey toward tranquility was marked by a deeper understanding of her fears and tailored interventions that addressed her specific needs. Anxiety in dogs, much like in humans, isn't just about visible signs such as trembling or whining; it's about understanding the underlying triggers that propel these behaviors. Hapa's triggers were not immediately apparent. It took keen observation to identify that loud noises, particularly thunderstorms, and the bustling energy of crowded places seemed to send her into a spiral of fear. Recognizing these triggers was the first step in helping Hapa navigate her world with less fear and more confidence.

Addressing canine anxiety effectively often requires a holistic approach—merely soothing a dog during moments of panic is akin to placing a Band-Aid on a wound that needs stitches. For Hapa, the combination of behavioral training to desensitize her to her fears, coupled with lifestyle adjustments that created a buffer against her triggers, laid the groundwork for her transformation. Desensitization involved controlled exposure to the sounds of thunderstorms through audio recordings played at gradually increasing volumes. During these sessions, Hapa's environment was made as comforting as possible, with her favorite blankets and toys close at hand, and treats were used to reinforce her calm behavior. This methodical exposure, coupled with positive reinforcement, gradually reduced her anxiety, making real storms more manageable.

Amidst these training sessions, adjustments to Hapa's daily routine played a pivotal role in managing her anxiety. Creating a predictable schedule is more than just a convenience for an anxious dog—it's a cornerstone of their emotional stability. For Hapa, knowing that she could expect a peaceful walk early in the morning before the streets got busy or that she would have playtime after meals helped establish a sense of normalcy and security. This predictable routine reduced unpredictable disruptions that could trigger her anxiety, providing a solid foundation of trust and safety from which she could explore the world more confidently.

Case of Transformation: Hapa's Newfound Peace

Hapa's story is one of many in the broader narrative of dogs overcoming anxiety, but her case stands out for the remarkable turnaround she exhibited. Hapa transformed from a dog who would hide at the slightest rumble of thunder into a more composed and joyful companion. Critical to this transformation was not just the desensitization and the routine but also the continuous support of her human family, who learned to scan her for signs of anxiety and intervene before her fears could escalate.

During a particularly challenging thunderstorm, after several weeks of desensitization therapy, Hapa could seek comfort without prompting. Instead of trembling beneath a couch, she fetched her favorite toy and nestled into her "safe spot"—a specially designed nook in her home filled with her blankets and a piece of clothing that smelled like her owner. This action was a significant milestone.

It showed that Hapa was not only learning to cope with her anxiety but was actively taking steps on her own to manage her feelings—a substantial victory for any dog dealing with anxiety.

Hapa's journey underscores the potential for transformation within each anxious dog. It highlights the importance of a supportive, patient approach that combines understanding the root causes of anxiety with practical, everyday strategies to reduce stress. Hapa's story is a testament to the resilience of dogs and the power of dedicated, compassionate care tailored to their specific emotional needs. It serves as a beacon of hope and a guide for others navigating the complexities of canine anxiety, proving that with the proper support and interventions, peace is not just possible but achievable.

A JOURNEY OF TRUST: REHABILITATING A FEARFUL DOG

The Impact of Fear on Behavior

Consider a dog like Tucker, a small Miniature Schnauzer, who would cower and whimper at the slightest sound, his body language spelling sheer terror. Fear, as seen with Tucker, can dictate a dog's interactions with the world around them. When dogs are fearful, their natural response can be to flee, hide, or sometimes show aggression as a defense mechanism. These behaviors are not acts of disobedience but rather survival instincts kicking in. For Tucker, his fear was not just an emotional response; it permeated his ability to function normally. He would often refuse to eat if there were too many people around, and loud noises would send him scrambling for cover. His quality of life was hampered by his pervasive anxiety, affecting his health and his ability to bond with others. It is crucial to approach such dogs with a strategy that acknowledges their fear without overwhelming them, setting the stage for a gradual recovery built on trust and comfort.

Steps to Building Trust

Building trust with a fearful dog like Tucker is akin to coaxing a wild bird to feed from your hand—a process that requires time, patience, and a lot of gentle encouragement. The key is to make every interaction predictable and non-threatening. For Tucker, this meant establishing a routine that he could rely on, where interactions with humans and other animals were controlled and always positive. The first step was to create a safe space for him, a quiet corner of the house with his bed and toys, where he could retreat whenever he felt overwhelmed. From there, trust-building exercises were introduced slowly. Initially, this involved sitting quietly near his safe space, speaking softly, and offering treats without making direct eye contact, which can be intimidating for fearful dogs.

Gradually, as Tucker began associating the human presence with something positive, these sessions would involve more direct interaction, like gentle petting or playful engagement with his toys. Each positive encounter slowly eroded his defensive barriers, incrementally building his confidence and trust.

Success Through Empathy and Understanding

Empathy in training means putting yourself in the paws of a fearful dog like Tucker and understanding that every loud sound or sudden movement can be perceived as a threat. Training methods for such dogs need to prioritize the dog's comfort and sense of security. Positive reinforcement plays a crucial role here, where desired behaviors are rewarded in a way that does not provoke fear. For instance, a soft tone of voice and gentle handling were employed instead of forceful commands or harsh corrections, ensuring Tucker felt at ease during training sessions. The focus was on making training a rewarding experience filled with many praises and treats, reinforcing his confidence, and associating new experiences with positive outcomes. This empathetic approach helps to replace fear with familiarity and anxiety with assurance, paving the way for a more relaxed and happier dog.

Real-Life Transformation: Tucker's New Chapter

Tucker's transformation was not an overnight miracle but proof of the power of patience and understanding. Over months of consistent and gentle training, the once-timid dog who would hide at every opportunity began seeking affection and companionship. One of the most heartwarming milestones was witnessing Tucker initiate play—a behavior he had never exhibited before. This breakthrough was a clear sign that he no longer viewed his environment as just a landscape of potential threats but as a place where he could also find joy and comfort. His journey, from a state of constant fear to one of curiosity and playfulness, was not just about teaching a dog new behavior but about giving him a second chance at life. Each small step he took towards overcoming his fears was celebrated, reinforcing his newfound confidence and reshaping his view of the world as a safe and rewarding place.

BREAKING BARRIERS: A DEAF DOG'S TRAINING TRIUMPH

When you bring a deaf dog into your life, you quickly learn that communication is not limited to the spoken word and the bond you build is based on trust, understanding, and alternative forms of communication. Deaf dogs, like any other dog, have the potential to lead whole and responsive lives—they interact with the world a little differently. Training a deaf dog involves tapping into senses other than hearing, primarily sight and touch, which can open a unique way to connect and communicate.

Overcoming Communication Challenges

The initial challenge with a deaf dog is overcoming reliance on verbal cues, the most common form of communication during training. The key is to develop a set of distinct visual cues or hand signals. These visual signals can range from simple commands like "sit" or "stay" to more complex instructions like "come" or "lie down." Each command is paired with a specific, recognizable gesture. For instance, a flat hand pushed down can signal "sit," while a sweeping hand motion towards your body might mean "come here." These signals must be exaggerated and consistent, helping the dog easily recognize and differentiate each one. Additionally, incorporating a vibrating collar that gently buzzes can help gain a deaf dog's attention without startling them. This collar acts as a nudge, a way to say "look at me" when they are not facing you, facilitating the beginning of a communication exchange.

Training Techniques for Deaf Dogs

Practical training of a deaf dog relies heavily on visual cues and touch. One fundamental technique is using a flashlight in low visibility conditions or at night. A quick flash can serve the same purpose as calling the name of a hearing dog, grabbing their attention back to you. During training sessions, maintaining eye contact becomes more important than it might be with hearing dogs. It keeps them focused and engaged, reinforcing that connection as you guide them through their lessons. Positive reinforcement remains a cornerstone of training, with treats, smiles, and thumbs-up replacing verbal praise. Every correct response to a command is immediately rewarded with a treat and a consistent visual or physical gesture of approval, such as a thumbs-up or a gentle pat. Over time, these positive reinforcements help build a deaf dog's confidence and assurance, validating their training and strengthening your bond.

The Bond Beyond Words

The relationship between you and your deaf dog might lack spoken words, but it is deeply founded on mutual understanding and non-verbal communication. This bond is intuitive, a connection that becomes almost palpable in its intensity. You learn to read each other's body language instinctively; a slight change in posture, the direction of a gaze, and the position of a tail can speak volumes. This developing silent dialogue is a beautiful aspect of living with a deaf dog. It highlights the unspoken power of companionship and love between humans and their canine friends, a testimony to their adaptability and resilience.

Celebrating Success

Take, for example, the story of Bella, a deaf Dalmatian who transformed from a misunderstood puppy into a champion in agility competitions. Her inability to hear did not hinder her; instead, it shaped a training regimen that was robustly visual and tactile. Her owner developed a series of hand signals that directed Bella through complex agility courses with precision and grace. Each successful run was celebrated with a shower of visual praises and treats, reinforcing her training and boosting her confidence. Bella's journey is not just the success story of a deaf dog excelling in agility competitions; it's a narrative that challenges preconceived notions about the limitations of deaf dogs. It is a powerful reminder of the potential within every challenge, the triumphs that can arise from understanding and adaptation, and the incredible, wordless joy shared between a dog and her trainer.

In training and living with a deaf dog, every small success is a milestone, a moment of joyous accomplishment that reinforces the effectiveness of patience, innovation, and empathy in overcoming communication barriers. These dogs teach us that understanding extends beyond words, that patience can forge paths where none existed, and that love, in any form, is a powerful language all on its own.

THE HIGH-ENERGY DOG WHO BECAME A CANINE GOOD CITIZEN

Meet Jasper, a whirlwind of fur and paws whose energy seemed limitless. For high-energy dogs like Jasper, it is crucial to find constructive outlets for their enthusiasm. These dogs often come from working breeds and possess a natural vigor that, if not properly managed, can manifest as destructive behavior or hyperactivity. The key is channeling this energy into positive activities that engage their bodies and minds. Structured play, agility training, and regular, vigorous exercise sessions became part of Jasper's daily routine. These activities did not expend his physical energy but provided mental stimulation, which is just as crucial for keeping such energetic dogs content and well-balanced.

Structured training sessions played a pivotal role in harnessing Jasper's energy. Training isn't just about teaching a dog commands; it's about engaging their mind to make them think, learn, and apply their learning. For Jasper, regular training sessions included obedience drills, trick training, and puzzle games that required him to solve problems to receive a reward. These activities made Jasper use his brain, reducing his restlessness by giving him a purpose and focus. The training sessions were kept short and dynamic to suit his attention span and to keep him interested and engaged. Consistency in these training sessions reinforced what he learned, ensuring the training had a lasting impact.

Achieving the Canine Good Citizen (CGC) title was a milestone in Jasper's life, marking his transformation from a hyperactive pup to a well-mannered dog. The CGC program is designed to reward dogs with good manners at home and in the community. The title recognizes a dog's obedience and demeanor and highlights the owner's dedication to responsible pet ownership. For Jasper, preparing for the CGC test involved mastering ten skills, which included accepting a friendly stranger, sitting politely for petting, walking through a crowd, and reacting well to another dog. Each task required patience and practice, pushing Jasper to focus his energy on specific behaviors and commands.

Jasper's journey to becoming a Canine Good Citizen is not just a story of training a high-energy dog; it's a narrative about finding balance and purpose. When Jasper finally passed his CGC test, it was a personal achievement for him and a moment of pride for everyone involved in his training. It demonstrated Jasper's ability to channel his energy into tasks that required concentration, patience, and calmness—qualities that were once foreign to his nature.

Jasper's transformation through his training and achieving his CGC title is a powerful reminder of what structured training and under-standing can do for a high-energy dog. It illustrates the potential within every spirited dog to find balance and purpose through guidance and training. Jasper's story is not just about a dog passing a test; it's about a dog enhancing his life and those around him through training and self-improvement.

As this chapter concludes, we reflect on the stories shared here and the impact that dedicated, empathetic training can have. Each tale illustrates the transformative power of understanding and patience. These narratives enrich our knowledge and deepen our appreciation for the resilience and capabilities of our canine companions.

The next chapter will explore specialized training strategies that can further enhance the skills and behaviors of dogs like Jasper, ensuring they succeed in their immediate environments and thrive in any situation. Continuing our exploration into practical dog training, we will look into the advanced techniques and approaches that can help any dog reach their full potential, reinforcing the themes of growth and achievement that echo throughout this book.

CHAPTER 8

BEYOND BASIC TRAINING

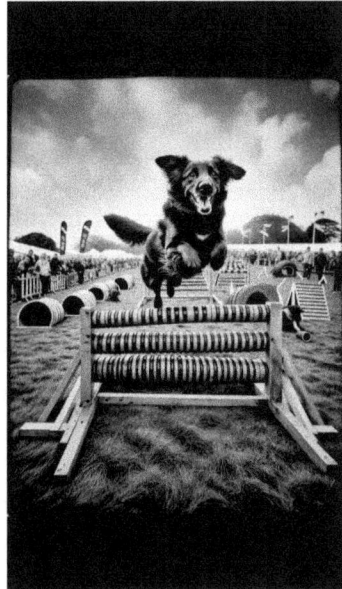

CANINE SPORTS: FINDING YOUR DOG'S PASSION

Have you ever noticed your dog's eyes light up at the sight of a frisbee or their tail wagging furiously as it races across a field? In these moments, the potential for enjoying canine sports becomes clear. Canine sports are not just activities; they are gateways to enhancing your dog's physical and mental well-being, offering you a unique opportunity to bond and explore new challenges together.

The World of Canine Sports

Canine sports are as diverse as they are thrilling, encompassing various activities that cater to different interests and capabilities. Agility courses, for instance, challenge your dog to navigate multiple obstacles like tunnels, weave poles, and jumps, all under the guidance of your cues. Flyball provides an exhilarating blend of speed and teamwork, where dogs race over hurdles to catch a tennis ball launched from a spring-loaded box. Then there's dock diving, where dogs take running leaps off docks into the water, competing for distance or height. These sports, along with herding, tracking, and rally obedience, stimulate your dog's body and mind and deepen your communication and trust.

Matching Sport to Dog

Choosing the right sport for your dog involves observing their natural inclinations and physical abilities. A high-energy, agile dog might thrive in agility or flyball, while an intense, focused dog might excel in weight-pulling or herding. It is also crucial to consider your dog's health; for instance, older dogs or those with joint issues might find swimming or nose work more suitable. Experiment with different activities to gauge what excites and engages your dog the most. It's also important to consider your interest and capability in participating in these sports. Remember, it's a team effort, and your enthusiasm is as important as your dog's.

Benefits Beyond Physical Health

The benefits of participating in canine sports extend far beyond physical health. These activities are potent mental stimulators, challenging your dog to learn new skills and solve problems quickly. This mental engagement can help alleviate common behavioral issues like boredom or anxiety by providing a constructive outlet for their energy. Moreover, the training for and participation in these sports strengthens the bond between you and your dog, built on mutual trust and the shared joy of achievement. This enhanced bond improves teamwork during competitions and enriches your everyday interactions.

Getting Started

Embarking on the canine sports journey is an adventure. Begin by joining local clubs or groups that offer training sessions. These groups provide valuable resources and support for both novices and experienced participants. They can offer guidance on training techniques, equipment, and even competition details. Many clubs also provide a community of like-minded individuals who can offer support, advice, and camaraderie, making the whole experience even more enjoyable for you and your dog.

Interactive Element: Find Your Dog's Sport Match Quiz

To assist you in determining which sport might be the best fit for your dog, consider taking an interactive quiz designed to match your dog's characteristics with a suitable canine sport. This quiz evaluates factors like your dog's breed, age, temperament, and physicality alongside your ability to participate and support them. By answering these questions, you can receive suggestions tailored to your unique situation, helping you make a well-informed decision about which sport to pursue.

Engaging your dog in sports is about more than physical activity; it's about discovering new ways to connect and communicate with your beloved companion. It's about watching them excel, sharing in their joy, and celebrating every achievement, no matter how small. Whether you're weaving through an agility course or cheering from the dock's edge, the world of canine sports offers something special for every dog and owner. So, explore these exciting possibilities and see where they might lead you and your furry friend.

DOGS GIVING BACK: VOLUNTEER AND THERAPY OPPORTUNITIES

Imagine your dog being your best friend and a beacon of joy for others facing challenges or simply needing a smile. Dogs have a remarkable capacity to give back to the community, serving in roles that touch lives and heal hearts. Whether visiting a hospital as a therapy dog, helping children improve their reading skills, or comforting those in stressful situations, dogs are uniquely suited to provide support and companionship where needed.

Roles for Canine Volunteers

The roles available for canine volunteers are diverse, each catering to different dogs' specific strengths and personalities. Therapy dogs are perhaps the most well-known; they visit hospitals, nursing homes, schools, and even disaster areas to provide comfort and companionship. Their presence can help reduce stress and anxiety, bring joy, and offer a comforting paw to those in need. Reading programs are another fantastic way for dogs to volunteer, sitting quietly while children read. This provides a non-judgmental audience to help boost the children's confidence in reading and nurtures a fondness for books and a sense of companionship. Dogs can also serve in more specialized roles, such as working in courthouses to provide emotional support to individuals during legal proceedings or in psychiatric units to assist those coping with mental health issues.

Training for Therapy Work

Training a dog to be a therapy animal involves more than basic obedience. While a solid foundation in basic commands is essential, therapy dogs must also be adept at handling various environments and social interactions. They need to be calm, gentle, and receptive to the needs of different individuals, often in busy or unfamiliar settings. Training typically includes exposure to various environments to ensure the dog is comfortable and behaves predictably in diverse situations. Additionally, therapy dogs must be screened for health and temperament, often involving evaluations by professional organizations certifying therapy animals. This assures the people involved that the dogs are not only safe but also effective in their roles.

The Impact on Humans and Dogs

The impact of therapy dogs on humans is well-documented through countless heartwarming stories and scientific studies. These dogs bring a unique form of therapy that can often reach places traditional methods cannot. They provide a sense of comfort, ease loneliness, reduce anxiety and stress, and even help with physical pain. The effects on the dogs are equally positive. Dogs are naturally social animals and often thrive on interaction and activity. The work gives them a sense of purpose and satisfaction, knowing they are making a difference. It also strengthens the bond between the dog and their handler, as they work closely together to navigate various social situations and help others.

Finding Volunteer Opportunities

Getting involved in volunteer or therapy work with your dog can begin with a simple search for organizations in your area that train and handle therapy dogs. Many hospitals, schools, and social service agencies partner with these organizations to provide programs. Additionally, reaching out to local libraries, educational institutions, and healthcare facilities can open opportunities that are not readily visible through larger organizations. Verify that any organization you work with is reputable and that proper training and support are available to you and your dog. This way, your interactions will be safe, positive, and beneficial for everyone involved.

Engaging your dog in volunteer or therapy work can be one of the most rewarding activities you undertake together. It allows you to give back to the community and helps foster a deeper connection with your dog as you work together to spread joy and comfort to those who need it most. Whether it's bringing a smile to a sick child, comforting a stressed-out student, or providing companionship to an older adult, your dog's roles in volunteering are as impactful as they are fulfilling.

THE WORLD FROM A DOG'S PERSPECTIVE: ENRICHING OUTINGS SEEN THROUGH THEIR EYES

Imagine for a moment that you're walking through a lush forest, but instead of standing upright, your eyes are just a foot off the ground, and your sense of smell is 40 times more powerful than usual. This is close to experiencing the world as your dog does. Dogs perceive their surroundings very differently from humans. Their color palette consists mainly of blues, yellows, and grays. They experience the world as a tapestry woven primarily of scents. Understanding these perceptual differences is crucial for providing your dog with experiences that are not only enjoyable but also engaging on a sensory level. Consider what your dog might find most interesting when planning outings—perhaps a trail with various wildlife scents or a park with diverse textures and shapes. You can turn a simple outing into a rich sensory feast that captivates your dog's attention and satisfies their innate curiosities by tuning into these details.

Designing Enrichment Outings

Enrichment outings are designed to stimulate your dog's senses and provide mental stimulation. Think of them as adventures that offer novel experiences for your dog to explore. Start by choosing environments that vary in landscape, smells, and sights. A beach visit, for example, introduces your dog to the unique textures of sand and saltwater, the sound of crashing waves, and the smell of seaweed. Forest trails offer different stimuli with earthy scents, the rustling of leaves, and the occasional squirrel darting up a tree. Even urban environments, with the myriad of human and traffic sounds and various visual landscapes, can be exciting for dogs if approached safely. To add an interactive component, you can create simple scent trails using safe, natural oils or treats, leading your dog on a treasure hunt that challenges their tracking skills and keeps them mentally engaged throughout the outing.

Safety and Preparation

Before heading out, take precautions for your and your dog's safety and comfort. Always check the weather conditions and avoid extreme heat or cold, which can be uncomfortable or dangerous for your dog. Keep your dog well-hydrated, especially if you're venturing out on warmer days, and consider bringing a portable water bowl. Check the environment for hazards such as toxic plants, unfenced cliffs, or overly crowded areas that might over-stimulate or stress your dog. It's also wise to update your dog's microchip information and ensure they wear a collar with an ID tag. For reactive dogs or those still in training, consider less crowded times and places or use tools like harnesses and long leads to give them freedom while maintaining control. Preparation is critical to making any outing successful so that you can focus on enjoying the experience rather than managing preventable mishaps.

Learning Together

Exploring new environments with your dog allows you to provide them with exercise or entertainment and share a learning experience that can strengthen your bond. Watch your dog's reactions and allow them to take the lead sometimes. This can help you understand their preferences and fears, allowing you to tailor future activities better to suit their personality. Use these outings to practice commands and reinforce training in different settings, enhancing your dog's adaptability and obedience. The more you explore, the more you learn about each other, creating a more powerful connection built on mutual trust and enriched experiences. These outings are not just walks or playtime; they are joint adventures contributing to a fuller, happier life filled with shared discoveries and joyful moments.

CANINE INTELLIGENCE: HOW DOGS THINK AND LEARN

The fascinating world of canine intelligence explains how dogs perceive, interact with, and understand their environment. Recent strides in animal cognition research have revealed that dogs possess a level of intelligence that mirrors that of very young children in many aspects. They can solve complex problems, understand numerous verbal commands, and read human emotional states. This cognitive ability allows dogs to engage in sophisticated forms of communication and learning, making them highly adaptable and capable companions.

Understanding how dogs process information is pivotal in optimizing how we train and interact with them. Dogs primarily learn through operant conditioning and observational learning. Operant conditioning involves learning through the consequences of actions, which is why positive reinforcement is so effective. On the other hand, observational learning occurs when a dog watches another dog or a human and mimics that behavior. It is part of beneficial situations where demonstrating a task is more effective than guiding a dog. For example, some service dog trainers use skilled "mentor" dogs to explain tasks to trainee dogs, who learn by observing and then imitating these actions.

COGNITIVE TRAINING GAMES

You can tap into and enhance your dog's cognitive abilities by integrating cognitive training games into their routine. These games are designed to challenge your dog and also to improve their problem-solving skills. Puzzle feeders, which require dogs to figure out how to access food by moving pieces or solving a puzzle, are a great starting point. These feeders stimulate a dog's brain and slow their eating, which is better for their digestion.

Another engaging cognitive game involves hiding treats around your home and encouraging your dog to find them. This game utilizes their natural scent-tracking capabilities and can be gradually made more challenging by increasing the number of hiding spots or masking the scent trails. For a more socially interactive game, engage your dog by teaching them to understand and respond to new commands or signals. Learning the command, practicing it, and being rewarded provide cognitive stimulation and build communication pathways between you and your dog.

UNDERSTANDING INDIVIDUAL LEARNING STYLES

Just as humans have individual learning preferences, dogs also exhibit unique styles and paces of learning, which can affect their training effectiveness. Some dogs might be motivated by treats (food-driven), others by affection (praise-driven), and some by toys (play-driven). Recognizing what motivates your dog is the first step in tailoring your training approach to fit their preferences. Additionally, the context in which dogs learn can significantly influence their responsiveness. For instance, a dog might learn more quickly in a quiet, familiar environment than in a noisy, busy park. Paying attention to these factors and adjusting training sessions accordingly can lead to more effective and enjoyable learning experiences.

FOSTERING INTELLECTUAL GROWTH

Encouraging continuous cognitive development in dogs enhances their learning capacity and promotes a healthy mental state, preventing boredom and related behavioral issues. Introducing new toys, games, and training exercises can stimulate and engage your dog mentally. It's also beneficial to rotate toys to maintain novelty and interest. Advanced training classes are another excellent way to foster intellectual growth. These classes offer structured learning environments where dogs can tackle new challenges and learn complex commands and behaviors.

Moreover, involving your dog in daily activities can provide informal learning opportunities. For example, asking your dog to help carry light groceries or to pick up their toys encourages them to apply their training in practical situations. This reinforces their learning and helps them understand their role in your shared environment, enhancing their sense of purpose and belonging.

By embracing the principles of canine intelligence, we open the door to deeper and more effective communication with our dogs. This understanding allows us to provide better mental stimulation, tailor training to fit individual needs, and ultimately enrich the lives of our canine companions. Whether through structured games, adaptive training methods, or daily interactive challenges, fostering our dogs' intellectual growth is a rewarding endeavor that strengthens the bonds we share with them, illuminating our beloved pets' profound capabilities and potential.

INNOVATIONS IN DOG TRAINING: TECHNOLOGY AND NEW METHODS

Just as with many areas of our lives, technology and innovative methodologies are transforming how we interact, teach, and understand our canine companions. Many tech tools and applications are available today, making training more accessible, efficient, and fun for dogs and their owners. Let's explore some groundbreaking tools and how they reshape the training landscape.

Tech Tools for Training

In dog technology, gadgets and apps can enhance the training process. Smart dog collars, for example, are a game-changer. These devices can track a dog's location, monitor their activity levels, and even provide insights into their health and behavior patterns. Some smart collars come equipped with GPS tracking, which is invaluable for the safety of dogs that might decide to explore beyond the backyard. Additionally, some collars offer training aids like tone or vibration signals, which can be used to communicate with your dog across distances, making it easier to manage them during off-leash activities.

Training apps are another fantastic tool that leverages technology for practical dog training. These apps often provide step-by-step training guides personalized to your dog's age, breed, and specific needs. They can include video tutorials demonstrating proper training techniques, ensuring you're executing the commands correctly, and using body language your dog can understand.

Furthermore, many apps allow you to track your dog's progress, schedule training sessions, and receive reminders for consistency, which is crucial in any successful training regimen.

Emerging Training Philosophies

The field of dog training is continually evolving, with new philosophies that emphasize science and positive reinforcement emerging regularly. These modern approaches focus on understanding the psychology behind a dog's behavior and using this knowledge to guide training practices. For instance, cognitive behavioral therapy, which has been widely used in human psychology to treat anxiety, is being adapted for use in dogs to help manage similar issues. This method involves altering a dog's response to certain stimuli through gradual, controlled exposure and positive reinforcement, reshaping their perceptions and reactions in a stress-free way.

Another innovative training philosophy is "consent training," where the dog has a say in the training process. This method teaches dogs to communicate their comfort levels during training sessions, promoting a more respectful and cooperative relationship between the dog and the trainer. It's a big shift from traditional methods that require compliance without considering the dog's willingness or emotional state.

Personalizing Training with Tech

Technology not only provides tools for training but also offers unprecedented ways to personalize the training experience. By gathering data on a dog's behavior, activity levels, and physiological responses, owners and trainers can customize training plans that cater to the dog's needs. For example, if an intelligent collar reveals that a dog is more active and responsive in the mornings, training sessions can be scheduled during these peak times to maximize effectiveness.

Behavior-tracking apps can help identify patterns that indicate stress or discomfort, allowing adjustments to be made before they become problematic. This level of customization ensures that the training is practical and enjoyable for the dog, leading to faster and more sustainable results.

The Future of Dog Training

Looking ahead, the possibilities for how technology could further enhance dog training are boundless. Imagine virtual reality environments where dogs are safely exposed to various stimuli, helping them learn and adapt without real-world risks. Augmented reality could one day allow us to see the world from our dog's perspective, deepening our understanding of their reactions and behaviors. AI-driven algorithms could analyze vast amounts of data from canine behavior, providing insights that could revolutionize training methods and canine communication.

Integrating technology in dog training opens a new frontier where the only limits are our creativity and innovation. As we continue to explore these possibilities, the future of dog training looks promising, with advancements that enhance the training process and enrich the lives of dogs and their human companions alike. These tools and methodologies not only make training more accessible but also more effective, tailored, and enjoyable, paving the way for a future where every dog can achieve their potential in a loving, understanding, and technologically empowered environment.

CREATING A LIFELONG LEARNING PLAN FOR YOUR DOG

The idea of lifelong learning for dogs is rooted in the understanding that, much like humans, dogs thrive on mental stimulation and challenges throughout their lives. This proactive approach to learning helps prevent the cognitive decline often associated with aging and keeps them engaged in their environment. This proactive approach to learning isn't just about teaching old dogs new tricks; it's about maintaining a level of curiosity and excitement that enriches their lives daily.

The Concept of Lifelong Learning

Consider lifelong learning as keeping the gears of your dog's mind well-oiled and operational. Dogs are naturally curious and intelligent creatures; without ongoing mental stimulation, they can become bored and develop unwanted behaviors. Continuous learning helps prevent these issues and improves their quality of life. Engage your dog in new activities, teach them new skills, and practice those they already know to keep their brain active and sharp. This isn't just about complexity or teaching progressively harder tricks but about variety and enjoyment—keeping the learning process fun and engaging for both of you.

Designing a Learning Plan

Creating a learning plan for your dog involves more than just a random selection of tricks and commands. It starts with setting achievable goals tailored to your dog's age, breed, and temperament. For a young, energetic dog, you might focus on physical activities that also require mental effort, like agility training or learning complex commands that require them to think and act. For older dogs, the focus might shift to gentler, more mentally focused tasks, like scent work or puzzle toys that challenge their mind without putting strain on their bodies.

This flexible training plan should allow adjustments based on your dog's progress and interest levels. It's also important to incorporate regular reviews of what's been learned, reinforcing old skills before introducing new challenges. This helps consolidate their learning and ensures they feel confident, which is crucial for maintaining their motivation.

Adjustments for Aging Dogs

As dogs age, their learning capacity and physical abilities change; the lifelong learning plan should reflect these changes. While senior dogs may not be able to perform physically demanding tasks, they can still engage in less strenuous activities that stimulate their minds. Modifying exercises to suit their comfort, like lower-impact versions of agility or short, gentle walks with plenty of sniffing breaks, can keep them engaged without straining their aging bodies. Additionally, cognitive games that require them to solve puzzles can help maintain their mental agility, combating the natural decline that comes with age.

Also, watch for signs of cognitive dysfunction, which can affect learning in older dogs. Symptoms like disorientation, atypical interactions with humans or other pets, sleep disturbances, and changes in activity levels can indicate cognitive issues. If you notice any of these signs, it's essential to consult your veterinarian for guidance on managing these symptoms and adjusting your learning plan accordingly.

Celebrating Learning Milestones

Recognizing and celebrating your dog's learning milestones is crucial for reinforcing their positive behavior and enjoying learning. Whether mastering a new trick, completing a challenging puzzle, or simply remaining engaged through a training session, each achievement is a step forward in their lifelong learning journey. Celebrations don't have to be elaborate—simple rewards like a favorite treat, verbal praise, or extra playtime can make a big difference.

Celebrating these milestones not only motivates your dog but also strengthens the bond between you. It shows your dog that you're paying attention and appreciate their efforts, making them more eager to participate and succeed. It's a beautiful cycle of learning, bonding, and mutual enjoyment that enhances your quality of life.

As we wrap up this chapter on creating a lifelong learning plan for your dog, remember that the goal is to teach, engage, and enrich. It's about creating a fulfilling life for your dog with new experiences and achievements. This approach to lifelong learning keeps your dog mentally sharp and physically healthy and deepens the bond you share, making every moment together even more meaningful.

SPREAD THE JOY!

No joy compares to that which a dog brings to your life, and the bond between you is one of the most memorable connections you'll ever make. This is your chance to get that gift to more dogs and their humans.

By sharing your honest opinion of this book and a little about your own experience with your dog, you'll help new readers find all the information they need to nurture a lifelong bond with their dog.

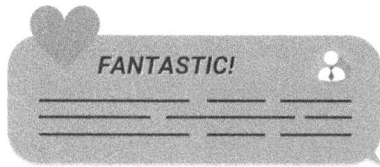

FANTASTIC!

Thank you so much for your support. I wish you and your dog all the happiness and adventures you desire.

SCAN ME

CONCLUSION

A Labrador Retriever made its way onto the platform of a local service station one day. He sat near the garage corner and began howling into the empty air. Weeks passed, and the dog would return every morning until the station owner closed shop in the early evening hours. Occasionally, the station owner fed the animal and placed a bowl of water for the animal to drink. One evening, the station owner attempted to take the dog home, but the animal resisted his prodding to get into the car. Curious, the station owner began asking customers about the dog.

The next day, a man came forward and claimed to know the canine's owner. The man said, "The master of this Labrador frequents your gas station. Unfortunately, a few weeks ago, he was involved in a serious car accident and could not locate this dog."

The stranger offered to return the lost dog to its owner. The stranger said, "The dog's master will soon be released from the hospital and is looking forward to reuniting with his furry friend." The Labrador willingly got into the strangers' vehicle and was returned to his owners' care. The highlight of this story is that dogs do not forget their master.

Moreover, they will patiently wait for their return.

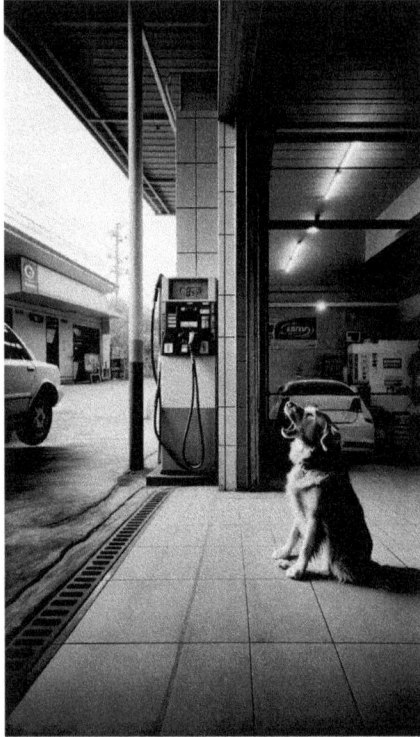

A dog has no use for fancy cars, big homes, or designer clothes; a water-logged stick will do just fine. A dog doesn't care if you're rich or poor, clever or dull, smart or dumb. Give him your heart, and he'll give you his. How many people can you say that about? How many people can make you feel rare and pure and special? How many people can make you feel extraordinary?

— (GROGAN, 2009)

As we draw the curtains on this journey through the pages of *The Human-Canine Connection: Enriching Your Life by Loving Your Dog*, I want to highlight your crucial role in this exploration. I hope you've discovered how deep and fulfilling the relationship between a human and a dog can be. Together, we've delved into the nuances of canine behavior, the effectiveness of positive reinforcement, and the continuous path of learning and connection that dog ownership entails.

Throughout this book, we've emphasized the importance of understanding, respect, and empathy. How we interact with our dogs can profoundly influence their behavior and emotional health. By embracing positive reinforcement, we promote better behavior and foster a secure and happy environment for our dogs. This approach isn't just about training—it's about building a foundation of trust and joy between you and your canine companion.

Dog ownership is indeed a lifelong journey. Each stage of your dog's life offers unique challenges and rewards, from the boundless energy of puppyhood to the gentle pace of their senior years. As we've discussed, adapting to these changes requires patience and empathy. It's more than pet care; it's growing together and deepening the bonds of companionship.

The role of proactive and informed pet care—through proper nutrition, regular exercise, and consistent veterinary checkups—cannot be overstated. These elements are vital for your dog's physical and mental well-being. They support your training efforts and ensure your furry friend's healthy, vibrant life.

Now, I urge you to put these insights into practice. Approach every training session, walk, and quiet moment of companionship with a sense of discovery and mutual respect. Celebrate the small victories, learn from the challenges, and always strive to see the world through your dog's eyes.

I also encourage you to share your stories. Whether it's a training breakthrough, a funny incident, or a moment of unexpected empathy, your experiences can inspire and support fellow dog lovers. By sharing, we can build a community of knowledgeable, compassionate, and supportive dog owners who value the deep connection of understanding our canine partners.

I want to express my deepest gratitude to you, the reader. Your commitment to learning about and caring for your dogs is commendable. Whether you are a new dog owner or a seasoned trainer, I hope this book has equipped you with the tools and knowledge to foster a relationship filled with respect, joy, and love.

May your days together be filled with wagging tails, wet noses, and that incomparable joy that only a dog can bring into your life. Here's to the beautiful journey ahead, shared with your loyal canine companions.

With warmest regards and best wishes,
Dwayne AJ Whogoes

REFERENCES

Smith, J. (2023). Revolutionizing dog training with modern technology. Today. Retrieved from http://dogtrainingtoday.com/revolutionizing-dog-training

Huffington Post. (2013). The dog was found guarding the owner's remains after Oklahoma. Tornado. Retrieved from https://www.huffpost.com/entry/dog-guards-dead-owner-body-oklahoma-tornado_n_3319239

The Arizona Republic. (2010). The dog keeps the child safe overnight in freezing temperatures. Retrieved from https://www.kold.com/story/12053880/dog-blue-rewarded-for-saving-little-girls-life/

Pet Science Daily. (2021). The science of petting dogs: How oxytocin bonds us *mentally* with furry friends. https://www.hopkinsmedicine.org/well ness-and-prevention/the-friend-who-keeps-you-young

Thorndike, E. L. (1911). Animal intelligence: Experimental studies. The Macmillan Company.

Five best techniques for aggressive dog rehabilitation. (2024, March 8). *Performance K9 Training & Boarding*. https://performancek9training.com/5-best-techniques-for-aggressive-dog-rehabilitation/

Armendariz, Y. (2022, January 2). *The ultimate guide to loose leash walking*. Canine Learning Academy. https://caninelearningacademy.com/dog-loose-leash-walk/

Bosch, G., Beerda, B., Hendriks, W. H., van der Poel, A. F. B., & Verstegen, M. W. A. (2007). Impact of nutrition on canine behavior: Current status and possible mechanisms. *Nutrition Research Reviews*, *20*(2), 180–194. https://doi.org/10. 1017/S095442240781331X

Burch, M. (2023, October 17). *How exercise can help improve your dog's mental health*. American Kennel Club. https://www.akc.org/expert-advice/health/dog-exer cise-mental-health/

Callahan, M. (2021, July 29). I am managing aggressive behavior. *Aggressive Dog*. https://aggressivedog.com/2021/07/29/managing-aggressive-behavior/

Chapagain, D., Wallis, L. J., Range, F., Affenzeller, N., Serra, J., & Virányi, Z. (2020). Behavioral and cognitive changes in aged pet dogs: No effects of an enriched diet and lifelong training. *PLoS ONE, 15*(9), e0238517. https://doi.org/10.1371/jour nal.pone.0238517

Clur, K.-B. (2022, November 27). Dog massage: Vet-approved techniques & how-to guide. *Dogster*. https://www.dogster.com/dog-health-care/dog-massage

Darling, N. (2023, January 23). *Don't confuse service, therapy, and emotional support dogs*. Psychology Today; Sussex Publishers, LLC. https://www.psychologytoday.

com/us/blog/thinking-about-kids/202301/dont-confuse-service-therapy-and-emotional-support-dogs

Does dog training work? A Success Story. (2023, April 10). Dog Gone Amazing Education Center. https://doggoneamazing.com/does-dog-training-really-work-a-dog-gone-amazing-success-story/

Gibeault, S. (2023, June 22). *Understanding dog body language: Decipher dogs' signs & signals.* American Kennel Club. https://www.akc.org/expert-advice/advice/how-to-read-dog-body-language/

Gibeault, S. (2024a, March 14). *How to stop your dog from jumping up on people.* American Kennel Club. https://www.akc.org/expert-advice/training/how-to-stop-your-dog-from-jumping-up-on-people/

Gibeault, S. (2024b, March 14). *Positive reinforcement dog training: The science behind operant conditioning.* American Kennel Club. https://www.akc.org/expert-advice/training/operant-conditioning-positive-reinforcement-dog-training/

Gibeault, S. (2024c, March 14). *Positive reinforcement dog training: The science behind operant conditioning.* American Kennel Club. https://www.akc.org/expert-advice/training/operant-conditioning-positive-reinforcement-dog-training/

Grogan, J. (2005). *Marley & me: Life and Love with the World's Worst Dog* (1st ed). Morrow.

How to stop a barking dog. (n.d.). The Humane Society of the United States. https://www.humanesociety.org/resources/how-get-your-dog-stop-barking

How to understand your dog's body language. (2024). Guide Dogs; Guide Dogs for the Blind. https://www.guidedogs.org.uk/getting-support/information-and-advice/dog-care-and-welfare/dog-body-language/

Karetnick, J. (2021, June 25). *How to train a therapy dog: Learning if your dog is fit for therapy work.* American Kennel Club. https://www.akc.org/expert-advice/training/how-to-train-a-therapy-dog/

Llera, R., & Buzhardt, L. (n.d.). *How dogs use smell to perceive the world.* VCA Animal Hospital. https://vcahospitals.com/know-your-pet/how-dogs-use-smell-to-perceive-the-world

Lowrey, S. (2023, May 26). *Why your dog needs a routine at every stage of life.* American Kennel Club. https://www.akc.org/expert-advice/health/why-your-dog-needs-routine/

Murphy, J. (2021, August 26). *Improve your dog's training success through play.* The Wildest. https://www.thewildest.com/dog-behavior/play-improves-dog-training-success

Revolutionizing dog training with modern technology. (2024, March 27). Gingr. https://www.gingrapp.com/blog/revolutionizing-dog-training-with-modern-technology

Reynolds, L. (n.d.). Benefits of training for dog sports. *Maximum Fun Dog Sports.* https://www.maximumfundogs.com/benefits-of-training-for-dog-sports/

Santo, K. (2020, May 27). *How to teach your dog scent work at home.* American Kennel

Club.   https://www.akc.org/expert-advice/training/how-to-teach-your-dog-scent-work/

Senestraro, A. (2022, December 11). *How can you tell if a dog is in pain, and what can you do to help?* PetMD; Chewy. https://www.petmd.com/dog/care/evr_dg_managing_pain_in_dogs

Small Door's Medical Experts. (n.d.). *Managing anxiety in dogs.* Small Door Veterinary.   https://www.smalldoorvet.com/learning-center/wellness/managing-anxiety-in-dogs/

Thomas, R. (2022, January 31). Mistakes using dog training treats. *Wellness Pet Food.* https://www.wellnesspetfood.com/blog/7-mistakes-people-make-when-using-dog-training-treats/

Thousand Hills Pet Resort. (2022, March 11). Five *benefits of clicker training.* Thousand Hills Pets; Son Care Foundation, Inc. https://www.thousandhillspetresort.com/post/5-benefits-of-clicker-training

Unveiling the genetics of dog behavior: Beyond breed assumptions. (2023, December 21). Stokeshire Designer Doodles; Stokeshire Media. https://www.wisconsindesignerdoodles.com/stokeshire-doodle-puppy-blog/does-breed-and-genetics-truly-impact-dog-behavior

Valentini, K. (2022, October 26). *Do dogs have emotions like people do?* Daily Paws; Dotdash Meredith. https://www.dailypaws.com/dogs-puppies/dog-behavior/dog-psychology/do-dogs-have-emotions

WebMD Editorial Contributors. (2023, May 28). *How to ease your dog's separation anxiety.* WebMD. https://www.webmd.com/pets/dogs-separation-anxiety

Weir, M., & Buzhardt, L. (n.d.-a). *Agility for dogs.* VCA Animal Hospitals. https://vcahospitals.com/know-your-pet/agility-for-dogs

Weir, M., & Buzhardt, L. (n.d.-b). *Signs your dog is stressed and how to relieve it.* VCA Animal Hospitals. https://vcahospitals.com/know-your-pet/signs-your-dog-is-stressed-and-how-to-relieve-it